**Echocardiography
Board Review**

Echocardiography Board Review

600 Multiple Choice Questions with Discussion

Third Edition

Ramdas G. Pai, MD, FACC, FRCP (Edin)
Professor of Medicine
California University of Science and Medicine
Colton, CA, USA
Chief of Cardiology and Director Cardiovascular Training Fellowship
Arrowhead Regional Medical Center
Colton, CA, USA
Professor and Chair Emeritus Medicine and Clinical Sciences
University of California Riverside School of Medicine
Riverside, CA, USA

Padmini Varadarajan, MD
Professor of Medicine
California University of Science and Medicine
Colton, CA, USA
Associate Program Director Cardiovascular Training Fellowship
Arrowhead Regional Medical Center
Colton, CA, USA
Professor Emeritus
University of California Riverside School of Medicine
Riverside, CA, USA

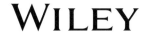

This edition first published 2025
© 2025 by John Wiley & Sons Ltd

Edition History
John Wiley & Sons Ltd (1e, 2008), John Wiley & Sons Ltd (2e, 2014)

The right of Ramdas G. Pai and Padmini Varadarajan be identified as the authors of this work has been asserted in accordance with law.

Registered Offices
John Wiley & Sons, Inc., 111 River Street, Hoboken, NJ 07030, USA
John Wiley & Sons Ltd, New Era House, 8 Oldlands Way, Bognor Regis, West Sussex, PO22 9NQ

For details of our global editorial offices, customer services, and more information about Wiley products visit us at www.wiley.com.

Wiley also publishes its books in a variety of electronic formats and by print-on-demand. Some content that appears in standard print versions of this book may not be available in other formats.

Library of Congress Cataloging-in-Publication Data
Names: Pai, Ramdas G., author. | Varadarajan, Padmini, author.
Title: Echocardiography board review : 600 multiple choice questions with
    discussion / Ramdas G Pai, Padmini Varadarajan.
Description: Third edition. | Hoboken, NJ : Wiley, 2025.
Identifiers: LCCN 2024041138 (print) | LCCN 2024041139 (ebook) | ISBN
    9781119812739 (paperback) | ISBN 9781119812746 (adobe pdf) | ISBN
    9781119812753 (epub)
Subjects: MESH: Echocardiography | Examination Questions
Classification: LCC RC683.5.U5 (print) | LCC RC683.5.U5 (ebook) | NLM WG
    18.2 | DDC 616.1/2075430076–dc23/eng/20241101
LC record available at https://lccn.loc.gov/2024041138
LC ebook record available at https://lccn.loc.gov/2024041139

Cover Design: Wiley
Cover Images: © kalewa/Shutterstock, © Panda Vector/Shutterstock

Set in 9/11pt PalatinoLTStd by Straive, Pondicherry, India

Printed in Singapore
M117228_251124

Contents

Preface

Echocardiography Board Review is written for the primary purpose of helping candidates prepare for National Board of Echocardiography and certification courses for cardiac sonographers. It should be helpful to both cardiologists and anesthesiologists preparing for this certification process. At the time of its initial writing there were no other published materials available that comprehensively dealt with the material covered in these examinations in a question, answer, and discussion format. The authors have used this format in teaching echocardiography to cardiology fellows in training. Part of the main impetus for initiating this book was the request by many trainees to write this kind of material. Similar requests also came from echocardiography technicians preparing for their certification examination.

There are close to 600 well-thought-out questions in the third edition of this review book. The questions address practically all areas of echocardiography, including applied ultrasound physics, practical hydrodynamics, imaging techniques, valvular heart disease, myocardial diseases, congenital heart disease, noninvasive hemodynamics, surgical echocardiography, and so on. Each question is followed by a number of answers to choose from. The discussion not only addresses the rationale behind picking the right choice but fills in information around the topic under discussion such that important key concepts are clearly highlighted. This helps not only in preparing for the test but also in promoting a clear understanding of various echocardiographic techniques, applications, and the disease processes they address. We have added separate sections dealing with adult congenital heart diseases and myocardial strain imaging.

This review will be helpful to not only prospective examinees in echocardiography but all students of echocardiography in training, not only in cardiology and anesthesia training programs in the United States but internationally as well. It does not take the place of a standard textbook of echocardiography but complements the textbook reading by bringing out the salient concepts in a clear fashion. The questions on applied physics, quantitative Doppler, and images are of particular value.

We feel this book will meet the needs of students of echocardiography not only in preparing for examinations but also in clearly enhancing understanding of the subject in an easy-to-read manner. The authors are grateful to the many trainees who expressed the need for such a work and pressured us to write one.

1

Questions

1. The speed of sound in tissues is:
   A. Roughly 1540 m/s
   B. Roughly 1540 km/s
   C. Roughly 1540 cm/s
   D. Roughly 1540 m/min

2. The relationship between propagation speed, frequency, and wavelength is given by the formula:
   A. Propagation speed = frequency × wavelength
   B. Propagation speed = wavelength/frequency
   C. Propagation speed = frequency/wavelength
   D. Propagation speed = wavelength × period

3. The frame rate increases with:
   A. Increasing the depth
   B. Reducing sector angle
   C. Increasing line density
   D. Adding color Doppler to B-mode imaging

4. Period is a measure of:
   A. Duration of one wavelength
   B. Duration of half a wavelength
   C. Amplitude of the wave

5. Determination of regurgitant orifice area by the proximal isovelocity surface area (PISA) method is based on:
   A. Law of conservation of mass
   B. Law of conservation of energy
   C. Law of conservation of momentum
   D. Jet momentum analysis

Echocardiography Board Review: 600 Multiple Choice Questions with Discussion, Third Edition.
Ramdas G. Pai and Padmini Varadarajan.
© 2025 John Wiley & Sons Ltd. Published 2025 by John Wiley & Sons Ltd.

6. In which situation can you not use the simplified Bernoulli equation to derive the pressure gradient?
   A. Peak instantaneous gradient across a nonobstructed mitral valve
   B. Peak gradient across a severely stenotic aortic valve
   C. Mean gradient across a severely stenotic aortic valve
   D. Mean gradient across a stenotic tricuspid valve

7. Which of the following resolutions change with increasing field depth?
   A. Axial resolution
   B. Lateral resolution

8. With a fixed-focus transducer with crystal diameter 20 mm and wavelength 2.5 mm, what is the depth of the focus?
   A. 40 m
   B. 30 mm
   C. 40 mm
   D. 4 m

9. A sonographer adjusts the ultrasound machine to double the depth of view from 5 to 10 cm. If sector angle is reduced to keep the frame rate constant, which of the following has changed?
   A. Axial resolution
   B. Temporal resolution
   C. Lateral resolution
   D. The wavelength

10. Which of the following properties of a reflected wave is most important in the genesis of a two-dimensional image?
    A. Amplitude
    B. Period
    C. Pulse repetition period
    D. Pulse duration

11. Increasing depth will change all of the following except:
    A. Pulse duration
    B. Pulse repetition period
    C. Pulse repetition frequency
    D. Duty factor

12. The two-dimensional images are produced because of this phenomenon when the ultrasound reaches the tissue:
    A. Refraction
    B. Backscatter
    C. Specular reflection
    D. Transmission

13. Attenuation of ultrasound as it travels through tissue is higher at:
    A. Greater depth
    B. Lower transducer frequency
    C. Blood rather than soft tissue like muscle
    D. Bone more than air

14. The half-intensity depth is a measure of:
    A. Ultrasound attenuation in tissue
    B. Half the wall thickness in mm
    C. Coating on the surface of the transducer
    D. Half the ultrasound beam width

15. What is the highest pulse repetition frequency (PRF) of a 3 MHz pulsed wave transducer imaging at a depth of 7 cm?
    A. 21 000 Hz
    B. 2333 Hz
    C. 11 000 Hz
    D. 2.1 million Hz

16. Examples of continuous wave imaging include:
    A. Two-dimensional image
    B. Volumetric scanner-acquired left ventricular (LV) image
    C. Color flow imaging
    D. Nonimaging Doppler probe (Pedoff)

17. Which of the following manipulations will increase the frame rate?
    A. Increase depth
    B. Increase transmit frequency
    C. Decrease sector angle
    D. Increase transmit power

18. The lateral resolution increases with:
    A. Decreasing transducer diameter
    B. Reducing power
    C. Beam focusing
    D. Reducing transmit frequency

19. Axial resolution can be improved by which of the following manipulations?
    A. Reduce beam diameter
    B. Beam focusing
    C. Reduce gain
    D. Increase transmit frequency

20. Type of sound used in medical imaging is:
    A. Ultrasound
    B. Infrasound
    C. Audible sound

Answers for Chapter 1

1. **Answer: A.**
Speed of sound in tissue is 1540 m/s. Hence, travel time to a depth of 15 cm is roughly 0.1 ms one way (1540 m/s = 154 000 cm/s or 154 cm/ms or 15 cm per 0.1 ms) or 0.2 ms for to-and-fro travel. This is independent of transducer frequency and depends only on the medium of transmission.

2. **Answer: A.**
Wavelength depends on frequency and propagation speed. It is given by the following relationship: wavelength (mm) = propagation speed (mm/μs)/frequency (MHZ). Hence, propagation speed = frequency × wavelength.

3. **Answer: B.**
Reducing the sector angle will reduce the time required to complete a frame by reducing the number of scan lines. This increases the temporal resolution. Decreasing the depth will increase the frame rate as well by reducing the transit time for ultrasound. Adding color Doppler will reduce the frame rate as more data need to be processed.

4. **Answer: A.**
Period is the time taken for one cycle or one wavelength to occur. The common unit for period is μs. Period decreases as frequency increases. The relationship is given by the equation: period = 1/frequency. For a 5 MHZ ultrasound the period is 0.2 μs (1s/5 million cycles/s = 0.2 μs).

5. **Answer: A.**
The law of conservation of mass is the basis of the continuity equation. As the flow rate at the PISA surface and the regurgitant orifice is the same, dividing the flow rate (cm^3/s) by the velocity (cm/s) at the regurgitant orifice obtained by continuous wave Doppler gives the effective regurgitant area in cm^2 (regurgitant flow rate in cm^3/s divided by flow velocity in cm/s equals effective regurgitant area in cm^2).

6. **Answer: A.**
In a nonobstructed mitral valve flow velocities are low. Significant energy is expended in accelerating the flow (flow acceleration). As the flow velocity is low, energy associated with convective acceleration is low. As viscous losses in this situation are minimal, the other two components (flow acceleration and convective acceleration) of the Bernoulli equation have to be taken into account. In the simplified Bernoulli equation, the flow acceleration component is ignored. Put simply, when you deal with low-velocity signals in a pulsatile system, the simplified Bernoulli equation does not describe the pressure flow relationship accurately.

7. **Answer: B.**
Lateral resolution depends on beam width, which increases at increasing depths. Axial resolution depends on spatial pulse length, which is a function of transducer frequency, pulse duration, and propagation velocity in the medium.

8. **Answer: C.**
Depth of focus equals squared crystal diameter divided by wavelength multiplied by 4. In this situation, $(20\,mm)^2/(2.5\,mm \times 4) = 400/10 = 40\,mm$.

9. **Answer: C.**
Lateral resolution diminishes at increasing depths owing to beam divergence. Frame rate determines the temporal resolution as temporal resolution is the reciprocal of frame rate. For example, frame rate of 50 fps gives a temporal resolution of $1/50 = 0.02$ s or 20 m. Wavelength is a function of the transducer frequency and is independent of depth and frame rate adjustments.

10. **Answer: A.**
Amplitude or strength of the reflected beam, and its temporal registration, which determines depth registration.

11. **Answer: A.**
Pulse duration is the characteristic of the pulse and does not change with depth. An increase in depth will increase the pulse repetition period, and hence reduce frequency and the duty factor.

12. **Answer: B.**
Backscatter or diffuse reflection produces most of the clinical images. Specular reflection reaches the transducer only when the incident angle is 90° to the surface, which is not the case in most of the images produced. Refracted and transmitted ultrasounds do not come back to the transducer.

13. **Answer: A.**
Attenuation is the loss of ultrasound energy as it travels through the tissue and is caused by absorption and random scatter. It is greater with longer travel path length as it has to go through more tissue. Attenuation is greater at higher frequencies due to shorter wavelength. Attenuation is greatest for air followed by bone, soft tissue, and water or blood.

14. **Answer: A.**
It is a measure of attenuation and reflects the depth at which the ultrasound energy is reduced by half. It is given by the formula: 6 cm/frequency in MHz. For example, for an ultrasound frequency of 3 MHz the half-intensity depth is 2 cm, and for 6 MHz it is 1 cm.

15. **Answer: C.**
The PRF is independent of transducer frequency and only determined by time of flight, which is the total time taken by ultrasound in the body in both directions. Ultrasound can travel 154 000 cm in a second at a travel speed of 1540 m/s. In other words, at 1 cm depth (2 cm travel distance) the technical limit to the number of pulses that can be sent is 154 000 cm/2 cm = 77 000/s (Hz). Hence, the PRF equals 77 000/depth in cm. For 7 cm depth, the total distance is 14 cm. PRF = 154 000 (cm/s)/14 cm = 11 000/s.

16. **Answer: D.**
Pedoff is a dedicated continuous wave Doppler modality without image guidance for velocity recording. All other modalities utilize the pulsed wave technique, in which each of the crystals performs both transmit and receive functions.

17. **Answer: C.**
Increase in the frame rate occurs by reducing the sector angle and reducing the depth, the former by reducing scan lines and the latter by reducing the ultrasound transit time. It is independent of transmit frequency and power.

18. **Answer: C.**

Focusing increases lateral resolution. Increase in transducer diameter and frequency also increases lateral resolution.

19. **Answer: D.**

Increasing the transmit frequency will reduce the wavelength and hence the spatial pulse length. This will increase the PRF and the axial resolution. Beam diameter and focusing have no effect on axial resolution.

20. **Answer: A.**

Ultrasound is used in medical imaging. The typical frequency is 2–30 MHz: 2–7 MHz for cardiac imaging, 10 MHz for intracardiac echocardiography, and 20–30 MHz for intravascular imaging. Ultrasound in the 100–400 MHz range is used for acoustic microscopy. Frequency >20 000 Hz is ultrasound. Audible range is 20–20 000 Hz and frequency <20 Hz is called infrasound.

2

Questions

1. Doppler shift is typically in:
   A. Ultrasound range
   B. Infrasound range
   C. Audible range

2. Duty factor refers to:
   A. Power the transducer can generate
   B. Range of frequencies the transducer is capable of
   C. Physical properties of the damping material
   D. Fraction of time the transducer is emitting ultrasound

3. Duty factor increases with:
   A. Increasing gain
   B. Increasing pulse duration
   C. Decreasing pulse repetition frequency (PRF)
   D. Decreasing dynamic range

4. Which of the following will increase the PRF?
   A. Reducing depth
   B. Decreasing transducer frequency
   C. Reducing sector angle
   D. Reducing filter

5. Persistence will have this effect on the image:
   A. Smoothening of a two-dimensional image
   B. Better resolution
   C. Eliminating artifacts
   D. Spuriously reducing wall thickness

6. Aliasing occurs in this type of imaging:
   A. Pulsed wave Doppler
   B. Continuous wave Doppler
   C. Neither of the above
   D. Both of the above

Echocardiography Board Review: 600 Multiple Choice Questions with Discussion, Third Edition.
Ramdas G. Pai and Padmini Varadarajan.
© 2025 John Wiley & Sons Ltd. Published 2025 by John Wiley & Sons Ltd.

7. The Nyquist limit at a PRF of 1000 Hz is:
   A. 500 Hz
   B. 1000 Hz
   C. 2000 Hz
   D. Cannot calculate

8. The Nyquist limit can be increased by:
   A. Increasing the PRF
   B. Reducing the PRF
   C. Neither of the above

9. The Nyquist limit can also be increased by:
   A. Increasing transducer frequency
   B. Reducing transducer frequency
   C. Reducing filter
   D. None of the above

10. Aliasing can be reduced by:
    A. Decreasing the depth
    B. Increasing the PRF
    C. Reducing the transducer frequency
    D. Changing to continuous wave Doppler
    E. All of the above

11. What is the purpose of the depth or time gain compensation process adjusted by the echo cardiographer and performed in an ultrasound's receiver?
    A. Corrects for depth attenuation and makes the image uniformly bright
    B. Eliminates image artifacts
    C. Eliminates aliasing
    D. None of the above

12. Which of the following increases the Nyquist limit?
    A. Increasing the depth
    B. Reducing the sample volume depth
    C. Increasing the transducer frequency
    D. None of the above

13. The maximum Doppler shift that can be displayed without aliasing with a PRF of 10 kHz is:
    A. 5 kHz
    B. 10 kHz
    C. Depends on depth
    D. Cannot be determined

14. The PRF is influenced by:
    A. Transducer frequency
    B. Depth of imaging
    C. Both
    D. Neither

15. Two identical structures appear on an ultrasound scan. One is real and the other is an artifact, the artifact being deeper than the real structure. What is this artifact called?
    A. Shadowing
    B. Ghosting

C. Speed error artifact

D. Mirror image

16. What is influenced by the medium through which sound travels?
    A. Wavelength alone
    B. Speed alone
    C. Both wavelength and speed
    D. None of the above

17. Image quality on an ultrasound scan is dark throughout? What is the best first step to take?
    A. Increase output power
    B. Increase receiver gain
    C. Change to a higher-frequency transducer
    D. Decrease receiver gain

18. All of the following will improve temporal resolution except:
    A. Decreasing line density
    B. Decreasing sector angle
    C. Increasing frame rate
    D. Multifocusing

19. Sound travels faster in a medium with which of the following characteristics?
    A. High density, low stiffness
    B. Low density, high stiffness
    C. High density, high stiffness
    D. Low density, low stiffness

20. Which of the following is associated with continuous wave Doppler compared to pulsed wave Doppler?
    A. Aliasing
    B. Range specificity
    C. Ability to record higher velocities
    D. All of the above

Answers for Chapter 2

1. **Answer: C.**
Doppler shift resulting from moving blood is generally audible as it is the difference between the transmitted and returned ultrasound frequencies. One can hear them during Doppler examination. Audible frequency is 20–20 000 Hz.

2. **Answer: D.**
It is pulse duration divided by pulse repetition period (PRP). Typical value for two-dimensional imaging is 0.1–1% and for Doppler it is 0.5–5%. Example for a 2 MHz transducer: Period = 1 s/frequency = 1/2 000 000 or 0.0005 ms. The wavelength in tissue is 0.75 mm (period = 0.0005 ms or 0.5 μs); if two periods are in a pulse then pulse duration is 1 μs or 0.001 ms; and if PRF is 1000 Hz (PRP will be 1 ms or 1000 μs) then the duty factor is 1 μs/1000 μs = 0.001 = 0.1%.

3. **Answer: B.**
Proportional to pulse duration if the PRP is constant. If pulse duration is constant, decreasing the PRF will reduce the duty factor by increasing the PRP. See explanation for Question 2. Gain and dynamic range have no effect on duty factor.

4. **Answer: A.**
Reducing depth reduces time of flight of ultrasound in the body and hence will increase the PRF. Transducer frequency, sector angle, and filter have no effect on PRF.

5. **Answer: A.**
Persistence is the process of keeping the prior frames on the display console and this will smoothen the image. This reduces random noise and strengthens the signal. However, fast-moving structures can produce artifacts and make the structures look thicker than they are. Some of the other smoothing algorithms include interdigitation and blooming to reduce the spoking appearance produced by the scan lines. Persistence does not affect resolution. It is a post-processing tool.

6. **Answer: A.**
Aliasing or wraparound occurs when the Nyquist limit or upper limit of measurable velocity is reached. The Nyquist limit is determined by the PRF. Spectral pulsed wave Doppler and color flow imaging are pulsed wave modalities.

7. **Answer: A.**
Nyquist limit = PRF/2.

8. **Answer: A.**
Nyquist limit = PRF/2. Hence increasing PRF will increase the Nyquist limit.

9. **Answer: B.**
Reducing transducer frequency will increase aliasing velocity and reduce range ambiguity. For a given detected Doppler shift, the lower is the transducer frequency, the higher is the measured velocity. V in cm/s = $(77\,F_d$ in kHz$)/F_o$ in MHz for an incident angle of zero, where F_d is the Doppler shift and F_o is the transmitting frequency.

10. **Answer: E.**
All of the above. Reducing depth reduces transit time and allows higher PRF. Also see explanation for Questions 8 and 9. In continuous wave Doppler there are separate crystals to transmit and receive crystals and hence no aliasing, thus allowing higher velocities to be measured.

11. **Answer: A.**
It is post-processing, which adjusts for loss of ultrasound that occurs at increasing depths.

12. **Answer: B.**
The Nyquist limit is determined by the PRF and PRF = 77000/depth in cm. Hence decreasing the sample volume depth will increase the PRF, which in turn will increase the Nyquist limit.

13. **Answer: A.**
The Nyquist limit is PRF/2. Hence a Doppler shift of >5 kHz in this case will cause aliasing. Depth influences the PRF.

14. **Answer: B.**
The PRF is influenced by pulse duration and time needed for ultrasound to travel in tissue. Increasing depth will increase the time spent in the body. Transducer frequency does not influence PRF but can affect Doppler shift.

15. **Answer: D.**
Mirror image artifact is a type of artifact where the artifact is always deeper than the real structure and occurs because of the structure or the surface between the two functioning as a mirror. The shape and size of the mirror image depend on the shape of the reflecting surface (plane, convex, or concave).

16. **Answer: C.**
Speed is determined only by the medium through which sound is traveling. For a given frequency, speed will determine the wavelength: the greater the speed, the shorter the wavelength. Period is the time taken for one cycle and is determined by frequency. Medium does not affect the period. Velocity = frequency × wavelength and period = 1/wavelength.

17. **Answer: A.**
The first best action to take is to increase output power. This will brighten the overall image. If the image is still dark, then the receiver gain should be increased.

18. **Answer: D.**
Multifocusing will decrease temporal resolution by decreasing the frame rate, whereas all the others will improve temporal resolution by facilitating an increase in the frame rate.

19. **Answer: B.**
Sound travels faster in a medium with low density and high stiffness.

20. **Answer: C.**
Aliasing and range specificity are properties of pulsed wave Doppler. Continuous wave Doppler is not associated with range ambiguity. Continuous wave Doppler will also permit recording of higher velocities than pulsed wave Doppler as it is not limited by the PRF since transmitted ultrasound is continuous.

3

Questions

1. As transducer frequency increases, backscatter strength:
   A. Decreases
   B. Increases
   C. Does not change
   D. Refracts

2. If an echo arrives 39 µs after a pulse has been emitted, at what depth should the reflecting object be on the scan line?
   A. 3 cm
   B. 6 cm
   C. 1 cm
   D. None of the above

3. The Doppler shift produced by an object moving at a speed of 1 m/s toward the transducer emitting ultrasound at 2 MHz would be:
   A. 2.6 kHz
   B. 1.3 kHz
   C. 1 MHz
   D. 200 Hz

4. In the example, the reflected ultrasound will have a frequency of:
   A. 2 002 600 Hz
   B. 1 998 700 Hz
   C. 1 000 000 Hz
   D. 2 MHz

5. Reflected ultrasound from an object moving away from the sound source will have a frequency:
   A. Higher than original sound
   B. Lower than the original sound
   C. The same as the original sound
   D. Variable, depending on source of sound and velocity of the moving object

Echocardiography Board Review: 600 Multiple Choice Questions with Discussion, Third Edition.
Ramdas G. Pai and Padmini Varadarajan.
© 2025 John Wiley & Sons Ltd. Published 2025 by John Wiley & Sons Ltd.

6. Reflected ultrasound from an object moving perpendicular to the sound source will have a frequency:
   A. Higher than the original sound
   B. Lower than the original sound
   C. The same as the original sound
   D. Variable, depending on source of sound and velocity of the moving object

7. Doppler shift frequency is independent of:
   A. Operating frequency
   B. Doppler angle
   C. Propagation speed
   D. Amplitude

8. On a continuous wave Doppler display, amplitude is represented by:
   A. Brightness of the signal
   B. Vertical extent of the signal
   C. Width of the signal
   D. None of the above

9. Doppler signals from the myocardium, compared with those from the blood pool, display:
   A. Lower velocity
   B. Greater amplitude
   C. Both of the above
   D. Neither of the above

10. Doing which of the following modifications to the Doppler processing will allow myocardial velocities to be recorded selectively compared with blood pool velocities?
    A. A band pass filter that allows low velocities
    B. A band pass filter that allows high amplitude signals
    C. Both of the above
    D. Neither of the above

11. If the propagation speed is 1.6 mm/µs and the pulse round trip time is 5 µs, the distance to the reflector is:
    A. 8 mm
    B. 4 mm
    C. 10 mm
    D. Cannot be determined

12. How long after a pulse is sent out by a transducer does an echo from an object at a depth of 5 cm return?
    A. 13 µs
    B. 65 µs
    C. 5 µs
    D. Cannot be determined

13. For soft tissues, the attenuation coefficient at 3 MHz is:
    A. 1 dB/cm
    B. 6 dB/cm
    C. 1.5 dB/cm
    D. 3 dB/cm

14. If the density of a medium is $1000\,kg/m^3$ and the propagation speed is $1540\,m/s$, the impedance is:
    A. $1\,540\,000$ rayls
    B. $770\,000$ rayls
    C. $3\,080\,000$ rayls
    D. Cannot be determined

15. If the propagation speed through medium 2 is greater than the propagation speed through medium 1 the transmission angle will be _____ the incidence angle.
    A. Less than
    B. Greater than
    C. Equal to
    D. Cannot be determined

16. If amplitude is doubled, intensity is:
    A. Halved
    B. Quadrupled
    C. Remains the same
    D. Tripled

17. If both power and area are doubled, intensity is:
    A. Doubled
    B. Unchanged
    C. Halved
    D. Tripled

18. Flow resistance in a vessel depends on:
    A. Vessel length
    B. Vessel radius
    C. Blood viscosity
    D. All of the above
    E. None of the above

19. Flow resistance decreases with an increase in:
    A. Vessel length
    B. Vessel radius
    C. Blood viscosity
    D. None of the above

20. Flow resistance depends most strongly on:
    A. Vessel length
    B. Vessel radius
    C. Blood viscosity
    D. All of the above

Answers for Chapter 3

1. **Answer: B.**
Higher frequency is associated with shorter wavelengths. Shorter wavelengths are more readily reflected compared to longer wavelengths.

2. **Answer: A.**
Ultrasound takes 6.5 ms to travel 1 cm in the tissues assuming a transmission speed of 1540 m/s. Travel time for 6 cm is 39 μs, hence the object is 3 cm deep.

3. **Answer: A.**
$F_d = (2F_o V \cos$ of incident angle$)/C$ where F_d is the Doppler shift, V is the velocity and C is the speed of sound in the medium. In this example, $F_d = (2 \times 2\,000\,000 \times 1 \times 1)/1540 = 2600$ Hz or 2.6 kHz. For each MHz of emitted sound, a target velocity of 1 m/s will produce a Doppler shift of 1.3 kHz. Angle theta or incident angle is zero; hence the cosine of that angle is 1.

4. **Answer: A.**
As the object is moving directly toward the source of sound, the reflected sound will have a higher frequency and will equal F_o plus F_d.

5. **Answer: B.**
The object moving away will produce a negative Doppler shift. Hence the frequency of reflected ultrasound will be lower than the transmitted frequency.

6. **Answer: C.**
As the cosine of the incident angle of 90° is zero, the Doppler shift is zero (see the Doppler equation in Question 3). Because of the angle dependence of the Doppler shift, the angle between the direction of motion of the object and the ultrasound beam has to be as close to zero as possible to record the true Doppler shift and hence the true velocity. Cosine of 0° is 1, cosine of 20° is 0.94, and cosine of 90° is 0. Angle correction is generally not used for intracardiac flows because of the three-dimensional nature of intracardiac flows and fallacies of assumed angles in contrast to flow in tubular structures such as blood vessels.

7. **Answer: D.**
Look up the Doppler equation in Question 3. Note that F_d depends on ultrasound frequency, velocity of motion, direction of motion, and speed of sound in the medium but not amplitude or gain.

8. **Answer: A.**
Amplitude is the strength of the returning signal. Vertical extent is the velocity of the object, and horizontal axis is the time axis and gives the distribution or timing of the signal in the cardiac cycle.

9. **Answer: C.**
Myocardium produces stronger or higher amplitude signals that have lower velocities compared to the blood pool.

10. **Answer: C.**
The blood pool signals have higher velocity and lower amplitude compared with myocardial signals. Thus, filtering of higher velocity/lower amplitude signals will allow only low velocity/higher amplitude signals that come from the myocardium.

11. **Answer: B.**
    The distance to the reflector is calculated by the range equation. The formula is ½(propagation speed (mm/µs) × round trip time (µs)). So solving the equation gives ½(1.6 × 5) = 4 mm. In other words, in 5 µs, sound would have traveled 8 mm (to-and-fro distance). Hence the depth is 4 mm.

12. **Answer: B.**
    The round trip travel time for 1 cm is 13 µs. Hence for an object at 5 cm, the travel time is 13 µs × 5 = 65 µs.

13. **Answer: C.**
    Attenuation coefficient in soft tissue is equivalent to ½ × frequency (MHz). In the above question ½ × 3 = 1.5 dB/cm. Multiplying this by the path length (cm) yields the attenuation (dB).

14. **Answer: A.**
    Impedance describes the relationship between acoustic pressure and the speed of particle vibrations in a sound wave. It is equal to the density of a medium × propagation speed. Solving the equation gives 1000 × 1540 = 1 540 000 rayls. Impedance is increased if the density of the medium is increased or the propagation speed is increased. Note that all units are in MKS (meter, kilogram, seconds). Hence the unit of rayls is $(kg/m^3) \times (m/s) = kg/m^2s$.

15. **Answer: B.**
    When the propagation speed in medium 2 is greater than medium 1, the transmission angle will be greater than the incidence angle.

16. **Answer: B.**
    Intensity is the rate at which energy passes through a unit area. Intensity is equal to amplitude squared. Hence if amplitude is doubled, intensity is quadrupled.

17. **Answer: B.**
    Intensity is given by the equation power (mW)/area (cm²). Hence if both power and area are doubled, intensity will remain the same, as both numerator and denominator are multiplied by the same number.

18. **Answer: D.**
    Flow resistance $= (8 \times length \times viscosity)/(\pi \times radius^4)$. Hence flow resistance is directly proportional to length and viscosity and inversely proportional to the 4th power of the radius.

19. **Answer: B.**
    Flow resistance decreases with an increase in the vessel radius. Refer to Question 18 for the relationship. Resistance to flow and hence flow rate for a given driving pressure depend upon radius, length, and viscosity.

20. **Answer: B.**
    Flow resistance is inversely related to the 4th power of the radius. Hence it is most strongly related to the vessel radius. $R\alpha\ 1/r^4$.

4

Questions

1. Volumetric flow rate decreases with an increase in:
   A. Pressure difference
   B. Vessel radius
   C. Vessel length
   D. Blood viscosity
   E. Vessel length and blood viscosity

2. Which of the following on a color Doppler display is represented in real time?
   A. Gray-scale anatomy
   B. Flow direction
   C. Doppler spectrum
   D. Gray-scale anatomy and flow direction
   E. All of the above

3. Approximately how many pulses are required to obtain one line of color Doppler information?
   A. 1
   B. 100
   C. 10
   D. 10 000

4. Multiple focuses are not used in color Doppler imaging because:
   A. It would not improve the image
   B. Doppler transducers cannot focus
   C. Frame rates would be too low
   D. None of the above

5. Widening the color box on the display will ____ the frame rate.
   A. Increase
   B. Not change
   C. Decrease
   D. Cannot be determined

Echocardiography Board Review: 600 Multiple Choice Questions with Discussion, Third Edition.
Ramdas G. Pai and Padmini Varadarajan.
© 2025 John Wiley & Sons Ltd. Published 2025 by John Wiley & Sons Ltd.

6. The simplified Bernoulli equation is inapplicable under the following circumstances:
   A. Serial stenotic lesions
   B. Long tubular lesions
   C. Both of the above
   D. Neither of the above

7. The Bernoulli equation is an example of:
   A. Law of conservation of mass
   B. Law of conservation of energy
   C. Law of conservation of momentum
   D. None of the above

8. The continuity equation is an example of:
   A. Law of conservation of mass
   B. Law of conservation of energy
   C. Law of conservation of momentum
   D. None of the above

9. Effective regurgitant orifice area by the proximal isovelocity surface area (PISA) method is an example of:
   A. Law of conservation of mass
   B. Law of conservation of energy
   C. Law of conservation of momentum
   D. None of the above

10. Doppler calculation of aortic valve area is an example of:
    A. Law of conservation of mass
    B. Law of conservation of energy
    C. Law of conservation of momentum
    D. None of the above

11. Calculation of right ventricular systolic pressure from the tricuspid regurgitation velocity signal is an example of:
    A. Law of conservation of mass
    B. Law of conservation of energy
    C. Law of conservation of momentum
    D. None of the above

12. Color flow jet area of mitral regurgitation depends upon:
    A. Amount of regurgitation alone
    B. Driving pressure and the regurgitant volume
    C. Presence of aortic regurgitation
    D. Degree of mitral stenosis

13. Factors influencing mitral regurgitation jet volume also include:
    A. Proximity of left atrial wall
    B. Heart rate
    C. Gain setting
    D. Filter setting
    E. Left atrial size
    F. All of the above

14. Amount of mitral regurgitation depends upon:
    A. Regurgitant orifice size
    B. Driving pressure

C. Duration of systole

D. All of the above

15. Hemodynamic impact of a given volumetric severity of mitral regurgitation (MR) is increased by:
    A. Nondilated left atrium
    B. Left ventricular hypertrophy
    C. Presence of concomitant aortic regurgitation
    D. All of the above
    E. None of the above

16. Which feature is consistent with severe mitral regurgitation:
    A. Jet size to left atrial area ratio of 0.5
    B. The PISA radius of 1.2 cm at an aliasing velocity of 50 cm/s
    C. Effective regurgitant orifice area of 0.7 cm²
    D. All of the above
    E. None of the above

17. When using a fixed-focus probe this parameter cannot be changed by the sonographer:
    A. Pulse repetition period
    B. Pulse repetition frequency
    C. Amplitude
    D. Wavelength

18. The following signal was obtained from the apical view in a 45-year-old man with a systolic murmur. What is the most likely origin of this signal?

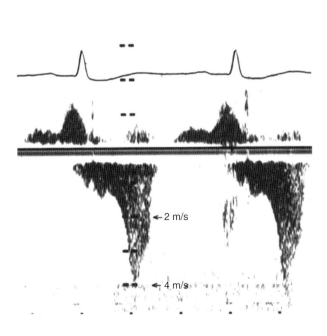

A. Mitral valve prolapse with late systolic MR

B. Rheumatic MR

    C. Hyperdynamic left ventricle with cavity obliteration

    D. Subaortic membrane

19. Continuous wave signal from the apical view. The image is suggestive of:

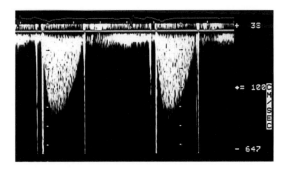

    A. Moderate aortic stenosis (AS)

    B. Severe AS

    C. Mitral regurgitation

    D. Prosthetic aortic valve obstruction

20. The signal obtained from the right parasternal (RPS) view is suggestive of:

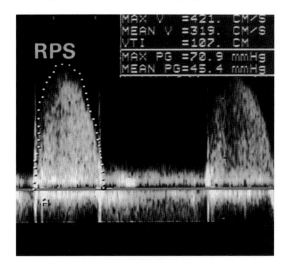

    A. Severe MR

    B. Severe AS

    C. Severe aortic regurgitation

    D. Severe pulmonary stenosis

Answers for Chapter 4

1. **Answer: E.**
   Volume flow rate = pressure difference $\times \pi \times$ diameter^4/128 $\times$ length $\times$ viscosity. Hence with an increase in length and viscosity, the volume flow rate will decrease. An increase in driving pressure and radius will increase the flow rate. Also, flow rate = pressure difference/resistance or pressure difference = flow rate $\times$ resistance (similar to Ohm's law of electricity).

2. **Answer: D.**
   Both gray scale and flow direction are displayed in real time.

3. **Answer: C.**
   Color Doppler is a pulse Doppler technique, and velocities at multiple depths along the scan line are needed to construct the color flow line. Using the multigate technique with placement of several sample volumes along the Doppler beam path, a 2D display of distribution of blood flow is generated. About 10 pulse packets are needed for each scan line of color Doppler to obtain precise information, as opposed to only one pulse packet to create one B mode scan line. Based on a propagation velocity of 1540 m/s, an echo signal reflected from a depth of 10 cm has a round trip time of 130 µs, which is the time required to generate a line of B mode scan. It takes 10 times longer, 1.3 ms, to generate a color Doppler scan line.

4. **Answer: C.**
   Combination of multiple pulses needed for a scan line, multiple focusing, and the need for some width for color flow display box will markedly reduce frame rate.

5. **Answer: C.**
   Widening color box reduces frame rate by increasing the number of scan lines per box.

6. **Answer: C.**
   For the simplified Bernoulli equation to work, the lesion has to be a discrete stenosis. In serial lesions there may be incomplete recovery of pressure and the flow area may be smaller than the anatomic area before the second lesion is encountered. Hence the pressure gradient at the first orifice estimated by the simplified Bernoulli equation will be lower than the actual gradient because of the unmeasured kinetic energy between two orifices. Thus the total gradient is not the sum of $4V^2$ at the two orifices. For long tubular lesions, viscous forces predominate and the Poiseuille equation would be applicable to analyze the pressure–flow relationship. The simplified Bernoulli equation does not apply to describe the pressure–flow relationship when the energy associated with flow acceleration is significant, as in a nonobstructed valve.

7. **Answer: B.**
   Describes the relationship between different types of energies as potential (pressure) kinetic (flow) and viscous forces along a flow stream. Energy can be transformed from one form to the other but cannot be destroyed or created.

8. **Answer: A.**
   Says that mass cannot be destroyed and hence flow rates at different locations in a flow stream are the same at a given point in time.

9. **Answer: A.**
   In the case of PISA, flow rate at PISA surface is same as the flow rate at the vena contracta. Flow rate is a measure of mass of blood transported per unit of time.

10. **Answer: A.**
    Based on the principle that flow rate at the left ventricular outflow tract is same as that of flow rate at AS vena contracta.

11. **Answer: B.**
    Is based on the simplified Bernoulli equation.

12. **Answer: B.**
    Driving pressure influences the jet area independent of regurgitant volume, as the jet area is proportional to the kinetic energy (KE) imparted to the jet, which is proportional to the jet, volume, and also the driving pressure (KE = ½MV² where M = mass of blood and V = velocity). Increase in driving pressure will also increase the regurgitant volume for a given regurgitant orifice. Hence doubling the driving pressure for a given regurgitant volume will double KE and jet size.

13. **Answer: F.**
    All of these affect the jet size. Compared to the central jet, a wall-hugging jet is about 50% smaller for a given volume (due to loss of kinetic energy due to wall contact) and a non-wall-hugging eccentric jet may be larger due to the Coanda effect where the jet spreads due to the pull toward the wall. Lower gains and higher filter settings reduce jet size. At a faster heart rate, due to reduced jet sampling the jet size may be underestimated. Free jet (receiving chamber at least five times the jet size) has a larger size compared to a contained jet entering a smaller chamber.

14. **Answer: D.**
    Regurgitant volume is directly proportional to the regurgitant orifice size, driving pressure, and the time over which regurgitation occurs.

15. **Answer: D.**
    Noncompliant left atrium as well as left ventricular hypertrophy will increase the hemodynamic impact of MR. Presence of aortic regurgitation will add another source of volume load on the left ventricle. Other factors that may have an adverse impact include anemia, fever, and acuteness of onset.

16. **Answer: D.**
    All of the above. Correlates of severe MR include MR jet area of ≥ 8 cm², jet to left atrial area of ≥ 0.4, vena contracta diameter of ≥ 7 mm, effective regurgitant orifice area of ≥ 0.4 cm² or 40 mm², and systolic flow reversal in the pulmonary veins. It has to be kept in mind that wall-hugging jets are smaller for a given regurgitant volume and the effective orifice area may not be constant during systole.

17. **Answer: D.**
    The wavelength cannot be changed by the sonographer when using a fixed-focus probe.

18. **Answer: C.**
    Left ventricular cavity obliteration. The thin dagger suggests a diminishing flow area in late systole. Although this can occur on left ventricular outflow obstruction due to systolic anterior motion (SAM), the peak tends to be a little earlier at this

gradient. A very late peaking signal is suggestive of cavity obliteration. This is a complete velocity profile and flow acceleration is clearly seen. In mitral valve prolapse, an incomplete signal may give a spurious late peaking signal. Signal profile depends solely on the left ventricular to left atrial pressure gradient in MR; only the signal intensity depends on the instantaneous regurgitant flow rate, which determines the number of scatterers.

19. **Answer: D.**
    Note the aortic valve opening and closing clicks. There are two opening clicks indicating dyssynchronous opening of a bileaflet mechanical aortic valve and a midpeaking systolic velocity of 4.5 m/s corresponding to a peak gradient of 80 mmHg. The gradient in the prosthetic valve depends upon valve size, valve type, and flow.

20. **Answer: B.**
    Severe AS. This is a signal occupying the ejection phase and directed to the right shoulder, which is typical of AS. A flail posterior mitral leaflet may cause a jet directed in this direction but is holosystolic starting with the QRS complex. The signal of aortic regurgitation is diastolic. The pulmonary stenosis signal is recorded best from the left parasternal, apical, or subcostal locations.

5

Questions

1. The Doppler signal is consistent with:

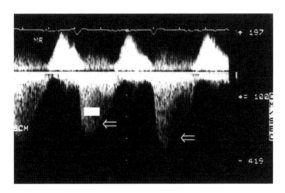

   A. Severe aortic regurgitation and moderate aortic stenosis
   B. Severe mitral stenosis
   C. Acute severe mitral regurgitation
   D. Ventricular septal defect

2. Pulse duration is affected by:
   A. Source of ultrasound
   B. Transmission medium
   C. Both of the above
   D. Neither of the above

3. The pulse repetition frequency (PRF) is affected by:
   A. Source of ultrasound
   B. Transmission medium
   C. Both of the above
   D. Neither of the above

Echocardiography Board Review: 600 Multiple Choice Questions with Discussion, Third Edition.
Ramdas G. Pai and Padmini Varadarajan.
© 2025 John Wiley & Sons Ltd. Published 2025 by John Wiley & Sons Ltd.

4. What happens to the PRF when imaging depth is increased?
   A. Increases
   B. Decreases
   C. Does not change
   D. Effect is variable

5. By increasing the PRF, the axial resolution:
   A. Increases
   B. Decreases
   C. Does not change

6. Imaging at depth affects:
   A. Axial resolution
   B. Lateral resolution
   C. Neither of the above
   D. Both of the above

7. Reducing the transducer footprint will affect:
   A. Lateral resolution
   B. Temporal resolution
   C. Axial resolution
   D. None of the above

8. Increasing the transmit power will:
   A. Decrease sensitivity
   B. Increase lateral resolution
   C. Increase penetration
   D. None of the above

9. Acoustic impedance equals (rayls):
   A. Density in $kg/m^3 \times$ speed of sound in m/s
   B. Density in $kg/m^3 \times$ transducer frequency in MHz
   C. Depth in meters $\times$ transducer frequency in MHz
   D. None of the above

10. Reflection of sound at an interface is affected by:
    A. Specific acoustic impedance
    B. Transducer frequency
    C. Depth
    D. None of the above

11. The most common cause of coronary sinus dilatation is:
    A. Heart failure
    B. Persistent left superior vena cava
    C. Atrial septal defect
    D. None of the above

12. The following data were obtained from a 72-year-old man with a calcified aortic valve: left ventricular outflow tract (LVOT) velocity (V_1) 0.8 m/s, transaortic velocity (V_2) 4 m/s, LVOT diameter 2 cm. The calculated aortic valve area (AVA) is:
    A. $0.4 cm^2$
    B. $0.6 cm^2$
    C. $0.8 cm^2$
    D. $1 cm^2$

13. The continuity equation is an example of:
    A. Law of conservation of mass
    B. Law of conservation of energy
    C. Law of conservation of momentum
    D. None of the above

14. The most practical value for the development of perfluorocarbon bubbles was to improve:
    A. Contrast on the right side
    B. Stable passage through the transpulmonary bed to improve contrast on the left side
    C. Improve contrast visualization in the hepatic bed
    D. None of the above

15. In a patient with mixed aortic valve disease, the AVA by the Gorlin equation using Fick cardiac output is likely to be:
    A. Less than by the continuity equation
    B. More than by the continuity equation
    C. The same by both methods

16. In a patient with mixed aortic valve disease, the AVA by the Gorlin equation using angiographic cardiac output is likely to be:
    A. Less than by the continuity equation
    B. More than by the continuity equation
    C. The same by both methods

17. The following measurements were obtained from a mitral regurgitant jet: radius of proximal isovelocity surface area = 1 cm, aliasing velocity = 40 cm/s. The peak regurgitant flow rate equals:
    A. 251 cc/s
    B. 251 cc/min
    C. 125 cc/min
    D. 125 cc/s

18. In the patient in Question 17, the systemic blood pressure is 120/80 mmHg in the absence of aortic stenosis and the left atrial pressure is 20 mmHg. The effective mitral regurgitant orifice area would be:
    A. 0.7 cm^2
    B. 0.5 cm^2
    C. 1 cm^2
    D. Cannot be calculated

19. This effective regurgitant orifice (ERO) area of 0.5 cm^2 represents:
    A. Mild mitral regurgitation (MR)
    B. Moderate MR
    C. Severe MR
    D. Severity cannot be detected

20. If the patient in Question 19 had a blood pressure of 220/90 mmHg with similar proximal isovelocity surface area (PISA) measurements, the ERO area would:
    A. Remain unchanged
    B. Be more
    C. Be less

Answers for Chapter 5

1. **Answer: C.**
   Acute severe MR. The image shows the classical "V wave cut-off" sign. The rapid deceleration of the MR velocity profile following the peak velocity is due to a rapidly diminishing left ventricular to left atrial (LV– LA) pressure gradient secondary to a large V wave in the left atrium that is a feature of severe MR, especially when it occurs acutely.

2. **Answer: A.**
   Source of ultrasound. Speed of ultrasound transmission does not affect pulse duration but affects wavelength. Pulse duration is determined by the transducer setting.

3. **Answer: A.**
   PRF is also a function of source of ultrasound and is not affected by medium of transmission. Speed of ultrasound transmission affects only lengths not the durations or frequency.

4. **Answer: B.**
   It decreases because of an increase in time of flight. PRF = 77 000/depth in cm.

5. **Answer: C.**
   The PRF does not affect axial resolution. Axial resolution is determined by spatial pulse length, which is mainly determined by wavelength (i.e., ultrasound frequency) and number of cycles in the pulse as transmission speed in biological systems is fairly fixed.

6. **Answer: B.**
   Lateral resolution drops because of beam divergence and widening. Axial resolution is unaffected by depth but is affected by wavelength (in frequency) and number of cycles in a pulse, which together make up spatial pulse length.

7. **Answer: A.**
   It will affect beam width and hence the lateral resolution.

8. **Answer: C.**
   Penetration increases due to more power. The sensitivity increases but lateral resolution decreases due to increasing beam width.

9. **Answer: A.**
   Acoustic impedance in rayls = density (kg/m³) × speed of ultrasound (m/s). Average soft tissue impedance is 1 630 000 rayls.

10. **Answer: A.**

11. **Answer: A.**
    Heart failure is the common cause of dilatation of the coronary sinus. Although persistent left superior vena cava (SVC) causes dilatation of the coronary sinus, it occurs infrequently. In the absence of heart failure, persistent left SVC is the most common cause of enlarged coronary sinus. Dilatation can occur either due to increased flow in the coronary sinus or due to increased right atrial pressure. The other causes include coronary arteriovenous fistula and unroofing of the coronary sinus. Unroofed coronary sinus results in a left to right shunt, a variant of atrial septal defect.

12. **Answer: B.**
The valve area can be calculated with the continuity equation. $A_1 V_1$ (LVOT area × LVOT velocity) = $A_2 V_2$ (aortic valve area × aortic velocity). $A_2 = A_1 V_1 / V_2$. $A_1 = \pi r^2$ (r = LVOT diameter/2) = $3.14 \times 1 \times 1 = 3.14\,\text{cm}^2$. $A_2 = 3.14 \times 0.8/4 = 0.6\,\text{cm}^2$.

13. **Answer: A.**
States that mass cannot be destroyed and hence flow rates at different locations in a flow stream are the same at a given point in time.

14. **Answer: B.**
The development of perfluorocarbon bubbles increased stable passage through the pulmonary bed, so that contrast visualization was better on the left side.

15. **Answer: A.**
The cardiac output by the Fick method is less than the transaortic flow, which is Fick cardiac output + regurgitant volume. Hence the calculation of AVA by Gorlin will underestimate AVA compared to AVA by the continuity equation. Gorlin equation will overestimate aortic stenosis severity.

16. **Answer: C.**
Angiographic and Doppler cardiac output would be equal.

17. **Answer: A.**
The regurgitant flow rate is calculated by the formula $2\pi r^2 \times$ aliasing velocity. This formula assumes a hemispherical geometry. Hence it is vital to optimize the aliasing velocity to maximize the hemisphere of the PISA in all dimensions. Using the formula, peak flow rate = $2\pi r^2 = 2 \times 3.14 \times 1 \times 1 \times 40 = 251.2\,\text{cc/s}$.

18. **Answer: B.**
The LA–LV pressure gradient is 100 mmHg, which corresponds to a peak mitral regurgitant velocity of 5 m/s or 500 cm/s. The ERO area is given by the formula $2\pi r^2 \times$ aliasing velocity (peak flow rate)/MR velocity. In this patient, peak flow rate = 251 cc/s and ERO is $251/500 = 0.5\,\text{cm}^2$.

19. **Answer: C.**
This patient has severe MR. The ERO is a fairly stable measure of quantitating MR as it represents the defect in the mitral valve co-aptation mechanism and is independent of loading conditions. ERO < 0.2 is mild, 0.2–0.4 is moderate, and ≥ 0.4 cm² is severe MR.

20. **Answer: C.**
Since the blood pressure is now elevated, the LV–LA pressure gradient is 200 mmHg, giving rise to an MR jet of 7 m/s. The ERO now is $251/700 = 0.3\,\text{cm}^2$. If the ERO were unchanged, the peak flow rate would be increased because of higher driving pressure and the PISA radius would be increased.

6

Questions

1. An intraoperative transesophageal echocardiogram (TEE) revealed mitral regurgitation with the following measurements: regurgitant jet area 4 cm², proximal isovelocity surface area (PISA) radius 0.8 cm at a Nyquist limit of 50 cm/s at a heart rate of 82 beats/min, and arterial blood pressure 80/40 mmHg. This represents:
   A. Mild mitral regurgitation (MR)
   B. Moderate MR
   C. Severe MR

2. For the patient in Question 1, if the systolic blood pressure is increased to 145 mmHg, assuming that the effective orifice area is unchanged, then the:
   A. MR jet size will double
   B. MR jet size will not change
   C. MR jet size will more than double

3. For a given regurgitant volume, all of the following result in a reduction in the jet size *except*:
   A. Fast heart rate
   B. Doubling the sector angle
   C. Increasing the imaging depth
   D. Increasing the blood pressure

4. In a patient with severe MR, all of the following factors increase its hemodynamic impact except:
   A. Mitral stenosis
   B. Left ventricular hypertrophy
   C. Compliant left atrium
   D. Concomitant aortic regurgitation

5. In a patient undergoing aortic valve replacement (AVR) for aortic stenosis, there was evidence of moderate MR on a preoperative transthoracic echocardiogram. After the AVR, the next step to be taken is:
   A. Replace the mitral valve
   B. Leave the mitral valve alone

Echocardiography Board Review: 600 Multiple Choice Questions with Discussion, Third Edition.
Ramdas G. Pai and Padmini Varadarajan.
© 2025 John Wiley & Sons Ltd. Published 2025 by John Wiley & Sons Ltd.

   C. Assess for MR with intraoperative TEE, and decide if repair or replacement is needed

   D. None of the above

6. A patient with old inferior wall myocardial infarction (MI) has severe MR with a posterolaterally directed jet in the left atrium. The most likely cause of MR in this patient is:
A. Flail posterior leaflet
B. Dilated mitral annulus
C. Tented or apically tethered posterior mitral leaflet
D. Tented or apically tethered anterior mitral leaflet

7. Presence of severe aortic regurgitation (AR) in a patient with mitral stenosis is likely to do the following to the calculated mitral valve area by the pressure half-time method:
A. Overestimate the valve area
B. Underestimate the valve area
C. No effect

8. Presence of atrial septal defect (ASD) in a patient with mitral stenosis is likely to do the following to the calculated mitral valve area by the pressure half-time method:
A. Overestimate the valve area
B. Underestimate the valve area
C. No change

9. In a patient with mitral stenosis, the following diastolic flow measurements were obtained: maximal radius of PISA 0.8 cm at an aliasing velocity of 50 cm/s, inlet angle 120 degrees, peak inflow velocity 2 m/s. The mitral valve area is:
A. 0.7 cm²
B. 1 cm²
C. 1.2 cm²
D. 1.5 cm²

10. A patient with mitral stenosis without any MR or AR has a stroke volume of 70 cc/beat and a transmitral flow integral of 50 cm. The mitral valve area is:
A. 0.7
B. 1
C. 1.4
D. None of the above

11. A patient with MR has a transaortic flow of 70 cc/beat by the left ventricular outflow tract (LVOT) method and a transmitral flow of 112 cc/beat by the mitral annular method. The time velocity integral (TVI) of the MR signal by continuous wave Doppler is 60 cm. The effective regurgitant orifice (ERO) area of this patient is:
A. 1.5 cm²
B. 0.7 cm²
C. 0.4 cm²
D. 0.2 cm²

12. For a patient with MR and AR, the following measurements were obtained using echo Doppler: flow across the pulmonary valve 75 cc/beat (no pulmonary regurgitation), flow across the mitral valve 120 cc/beat, flow across the aortic valve 90 cc/beat, TVI of MR signal 90 cm, TVI of AR signal 75 cm. The following statement is accurate in this patient:
    A. MR ERO is 0.5 cm² and AR ERO is 0.2 cm²
    B. MR ERO is 1.3 cm² and AR ERO is 1.2 cm²
    C. Cannot be calculated

13. In a patient with isolated AR, the following measurements were obtained: transmitral flow 80 cc/beat, flow across aortic valve 140 cc/beat, TVI of AR signal 100 cm. The AR in this patient is:
    A. Mild
    B. Moderate
    C. Severe
    D. Cannot be determined

14. A patient with dilated cardiomyopathy has an end diastolic pulmonary regurgitation (PR) velocity of 2 m/s and the estimated right atrial pressure is 10 mmHg. The following statement is true about this patient:
    A. Pulmonary artery (PA) pressure is normal
    B. Has mild or moderate pulmonary hypertension
    C. Has severe pulmonary hypertension
    D. Cannot estimate pulmonary pressure

15. If the patient in Question 14 had valvular pulmonary stenosis (PS) with a peak gradient of 36 mmHg, the estimated PA end diastolic pressure would be:
    A. 16 mmHg
    B. 26 mmHg
    C. 36 mmHg
    D. 62 mmHg

16. If the patient in Question 14 has tricuspid stenosis with a mean diastolic gradient of 8 mmHg across the tricuspid valve, the PA diastolic pressure would be:
    A. 26 mmHg
    B. 34 mmHg
    C. 18 mmHg
    D. Cannot be estimated

17. In a patient with valvular PS with right PA branch stenosis, the following measurements were obtained: tricuspid regurgitation (TR) velocity 4 m/s, right atrial (RA) pressure 6 mmHg, systolic velocity across the pulmonary valve 2.5 m/s, velocity across the discrete branch stenosis 2.5 m/s. The systolic pressure in the right pulmonary branch distal to the stenosis is likely to be:
    A. 20 mmHg
    B. 5 mmHg
    C. 70 mmHg
    D. Cannot be estimated

18. A 20-year-old patient with a large ventricular septal defect (VSD) underwent PA banding in childhood and was lost to follow-up. A recent echocardiogram revealed the following: peak systolic velocity across the VSD 3 m/s, TR velocity 5 m/s, estimated RA pressure 10 mmHg, cuff blood pressure in the right arm 146/70 mmHg, peak flow velocity across the pulmonary band 4.7 m/s. The following statement is true:
    A. This patient has normal PA pressure
    B. The patient has severe pulmonary hypertension
    C. The patient has features of left ventricular (LV) failure
    D. PA pressure cannot be determined

19. The patient has an LVOT velocity of 1 m/s, velocity time integral (VTI) of 25 cm, LVOT diameter of 2 cm, aortic transvalvular velocity of 1.5 m/s, heart rate of 70 beats/min, and the cardiac output in this patient is:
    A. 5.5 L
    B. 4.5 L
    C. 6.3 L
    D. Cannot be determined based on the given data

20. A patient with aortic stenosis has an LVOT diameter of 2 cm, LVOT velocity (V_1) of 2.5 m/s, transaortic valve velocity (V_2) of 5 m/s, and two-dimensional examination showed moderate systolic anterior motion of the mitral leaflet. Valvular aortic stenosis in this patient is:
    A. Mild
    B. Moderate
    C. Severe
    D. Cannot be calculated based on the given data

Answers for Chapter 6

1. **Answer: C.**
Jet area underestimates the severity of MR as the driving pressure is low. The regurgitant flow rate is approximately 200 cc/s. Because of low left ventricular (LV) systolic pressure of 80 mmHg, the MR velocity would be in the range of 4 m/s (400 cm/s) assuming an left atrial (LA) pressure of 16 mmHg. Hence, the ERO area would be about 200/400 or 0.5 cm². Thus in an intraoperative setting, it is important to bring up the blood pressure before performing MR quantitation.

2. **Answer: C.**
As the driving pressure across the mitral valve is doubled, the regurgitant volume is doubled, as it is directly proportional to the driving pressure. However, jet size is not only dependent on regurgitant volume but also on the kinetic energy imparted to the jet, which depends on jet velocity and, indirectly, the driving pressure, kinetic energy = ½MV². In this patient the jet area would be theoretically about four times larger – that is, 16 cm² – as both regurgitant mass and driving pressure have doubled. However, the constraining effect of the left atrium will make it slightly smaller.

3. **Answer: D.**
Underestimation of MR can occur due to undersampling in the setting of low frame rate (increasing sector angle and depth) and high heart rates. Increasing blood pressure will increase the driving pressure across the mitral valve and hence the jet size will increase.

4. **Answer: C.**
A noncompliant left atrium causes a greater rise in left atrial pressure for a given regurgitant volume as it occurs in acute MR. Noncompliant left ventricle and concomitant volume overloads such as aortic regurgitation and anemia increase LV diastolic pressure. In patients with mitral stenosis, the presence of MR increases the transvalvular flow and the gradient.

5. **Answer: C.**
This patient had evidence of moderate MR on the preoperative echocardiogram. In most patients, just replacing the aortic valve causes MR to regress. The MR, if functional, regresses with AVR, but MR due to structural pathology is unlikely to regress. The functional MR is due to high driving pressure and increased LV end systolic size. With the relief of the high driving pressure, it is likely to regress. But after the AVR, the mitral valve should be assessed intraoperatively to decide if there is a need to address MR. There is no clear consensus on decision-making in patients like these.

6. **Answer: C.**
In a patient with inferior MI, a posterolateral MR jet can occur due to tented posterior leaflet or flail anterior leaflet. In this patient with inferior MI, the likely mechanism of MR is posterolateral displacement of papillary muscle causing apical tethering of posterior mitral leaflet, especially P2 and P3 segments. This jet would be posteriorly directed and originates at the medial commissure.

7. **Answer: A.**
In the presence of severe AR, the mitral pressure half-time is decreased due to a rise in LV diastolic pressure produced by AR. Hence, in the calculation of mitral valve area by the pressure half-time method, the valve area will be overestimated or mitral stenosis severity will be underestimated. Pressure half-time is decreased due to increase in late left ventricular diastolic pressure, causing a reduction in the LA–LV pressure gradient.

8. **Answer: A.**
ASD will cause left atrial decompression, and hence would result in rapid reduction in the LA–LV diastolic gradient through diastole, decreasing the pressure half-time. This will cause overestimation of the mitral valve area or underestimation of mitral stenosis severity.

9. **Answer: A.**
The peak inflow rate has to be corrected for the inlet angle as the shape of the PISA is not hemispheric but two-thirds of a hemisphere. Hence the peak flow rate is given by the formula $2 \times 3.14 \times r^2 \times$ (angle of inlet/180) $\times$ aliasing velocity. By this formula, the flow rate divided by the peak inflow velocity in cm/s gives the mitral valve area in cm². MVA = $\{2 \times 3.14 \times (0.8^2) \times (120/180)\}/200 = 0.7$ cm².

10. **Answer: C.**
The transmitral flow volume per beat would be the same as the stroke volume, that is, 70 cc/beat (70 cm³/beat). In the absence of MR, the effective diastolic mitral orifice area would be 70 cm³/50 cm = 1.4 cm².

11. **Answer: B.**
The effective regurgitant volume is 42 cm³ (112 − 70). The ERO area is the effective regurgitant volume (cm³)/TVI of MR signal (cm). Hence, 42/60 = 0.7 cm². The ERO area is 0.7 cm². Note the units of each of the measurements; in addition, the flow rate is in cm³/s. Paying attention to these is helpful in formulating the various equations. For example, the ERO area can also be obtained by dividing the peak regurgitant flow rate obtained by the PISA method (which is in cm³/s) by the peak regurgitant velocity (which is in cm/s) such that the unit of measurement remains in cm².

12. **Answer. A.**
The true forward stroke volume is 75 cc/beat, in the absence of pulmonary regurgitation. Mitral regurgitant volume is 120 − 75 = 45 cc and aortic regurgitant volume is 90 − 75 = 15 cc. Dividing the regurgitant volume by their respective TVIs will yield their effective regurgitant orifice area.

13. **Answer. C.**
Regurgitant volume is 140 − 80 = 60 cc/beat and regurgitant fraction is 60/140 = 44%. Effective regurgitant orifice area is regurgitant volume/TVI of aortic signal, that is, 60/100 = 0.6 cm². The regurgitant fraction in AR depends not only on ERO but on diastolic period and driving pressure. Hence, the ERO area is a more reliable index of AR volumetric severity. An ERO area of ≥ 0.3 cm² is indicative of severe AR.

14. **Answer: B.**
End diastolic PR velocity of 2 m/s represents a PA–RV (right ventricular) end diastolic gradient of 16 mmHg. Assuming an RV end diastolic pressure of 10 mmHg (same as RA pressure), the PA diastolic pressure will be 26 mmHg, which is in the moderate range.

15. **Answer: B.**
Systolic gradient across the pulmonary valve does not affect the diastolic pressure gradient based on the simplified Bernoulli equation. The only two determinants of PA end diastolic pressure are the PA–RV end diastolic gradient and the RV end diastolic pressure, which is assumed to be equal to the RA pressure.

16. **Answer: C.**
In this patient, RV end diastolic pressure equals RA pressure – tricuspid stenosis diastolic gradient $(10-8=2\,mmHg)$. The PA end diastolic pressure will be $16+2=18\,mmHg$.

17. **Answer: A.**
In this patient the estimated right ventricular systolic pressure (RVSP) is $64+6\,mmHg=70\,mmHg$. Pressure drop across the pulmonary valve is equal to $25\,mmHg$, resulting in a systolic pressure of $45\,mmHg$ in the main PA. As there is 3–4 cm between the pulmonary valve and the right PA, flow streams would have normalized and would allow us to estimate the pressure drop at the branch stenosis without the limitations of stenosis in series, unless there is a substantial pressure recovery. As the pressure drop across the branch stenosis is $25\,mmHg$, estimated systolic pressure distal to the branch stenosis is $45-25$ or $20\,mmHg$.

18. **Answer: A.**
The RV systolic pressure is $110\,mmHg$ based on TR velocity $(5\times5\times4+10=110\,mmHg)$. VSD peak velocity is $3\,m/s$ corresponding to an LV–RV pressure gradient of $36\,mmHg$. Given the systemic systolic pressure of $146\,mmHg$ (hence an LV systolic pressure of $146\,mmHg$), the VSD gradient is again concordant with an RV systolic pressure of $110\,mmHg$. In the absence of PS, this is the pressure in the proximal PA. The pressure gradient across the band is $4.7\times4.7\times4=88\,mmHg$. Hence the PA systolic pressure distal to the band is $110-88=22\,mmHg$. Although technically this patient has severe elevation of proximal PA pressure, the PA vascular perfusion pressure is normal, indicating the absence of pulmonary arterial disease, making this patient a candidate for surgical closure of VSD.

19. **Answer: A.**
The stroke volume equals the cross-sectional area $\times$ TVI of LVOT, which is $3.14\times1\times1\times25=78\,cc$. Stroke volume multiplied by heart rate, that is, $78\times70=5.5\,L/min$, equals cardiac output.

20. **Answer: D.**
In a patient with serial stenosis in close proximity, the continuity equation cannot be applied because of difficulty in obtaining precise subvalvular velocity and cross-sectional area of the flow in the LVOT. In a person without systolic anterior motion the cross-sectional area of subvalvular flow is roughly equal to the cross-sectional area of the LV outflow tract. Subvalvular obstruction will result in flow streams such that the cross-sectional area of flow is less than the anatomic LVOT area.

Questions

1. Bicuspid aortic valve may be associated with:
   A. Coronary anomalies
   B. Coarctation of the aorta
   C. Atrial septal defect
   D. None of the above

2. A dilated coronary sinus could be seen in all of the following conditions except:
   A. Right atrial hypertension
   B. Persistent left superior vena cava
   C. Coronary A–V fistula
   D. Unroofed coronary sinus
   E. Azygos continuity of inferior vena cava

3. Atrial septal defect (ASD) of sinus venosus type is most commonly associated with:
   A. Anomalous drainage of right upper pulmonary vein into the right atrium
   B. Anomalous drainage of left upper pulmonary vein into the right atrium
   C. Persistent left upper superior vena cava
   D. Coronary artery anomalies

4. Ostium primum ASD is most commonly associated with:
   A. Cleft in anterior mitral leaflet
   B. Cleft in septal leaflet of the tricuspid valve
   C. Patent ductus arteriosus
   D. Aortic stenosis

5. Dilatation of the pulmonary artery is seen in all of the following conditions except:
   A. Atrial septal defect
   B. Valvular pulmonary stenosis
   C. Infundibular pulmonary stenosis
   D. Pulmonary hypertension

Echocardiography Board Review: 600 Multiple Choice Questions with Discussion, Third Edition.
Ramdas G. Pai and Padmini Varadarajan.
© 2025 John Wiley & Sons Ltd. Published 2025 by John Wiley & Sons Ltd.

6. Risk of aortic dissection is increased in the following conditions except:
   A. Marfan's syndrome
   B. Bicuspid aortic valve
   C. Pregnancy
   D. Mitral stenosis

7. A 52-year-old patient with a 31 mm St. Jude mitral valve has severe shortness of breath. Left ventricular function and aortic valve are normal. The disk motion of the prosthetic valve is normal. Analysis of transmitral flow with continuous wave Doppler revealed an E-wave velocity of 2.6 m/s, A-wave velocity of 0.6 m/s, E-wave pressure half-time of 40 ms, diastolic mean gradient of 6 mmHg at a heart rate of 60/min, and isovolumic relaxation time (IVRT) of 30 ms. This patient is likely to have:
   A. Mitral regurgitation
   B. Pannus growth into the prosthetic valve
   C. Prosthetic valve thrombosis
   D. Normal prosthetic valve function

8. In a person with suspected paravalvular (mechanical) mitral regurgitation (MR), the following transducer position has the best chance of revealing the MR jet:
   A. Parasternal long axis view
   B. Apical four-chamber
   C. Apical two-chamber
   D. Apical long axis

9. A patient with a bileaflet mechanical aortic valve has shortness of breath on exertion. An echocardiogram revealed normal left ventricular systolic function and mitral valve function. The left ventricular outflow tract (LVOT) dimension was 2.2 cm, LVOT (V_1) velocity was 1.5 m/s, and aortic transvalvular velocity (V_2) was 4.5 m/s, with no aortic regurgitation. Measurements obtained 2 years earlier when the patient was asymptomatic were LVOT diameter 2.2 cm, V_1 0.9 m/s, and V_2 2.7 m/s. Likely cause of this patient's shortness of breath is:
   A. Prosthetic valve stenosis
   B. Patient–prosthesis mismatch
   C. High cardiac output state, patient may be anemic
   D. None of the above

10. A patient with a mechanical prosthetic mitral valve has gastrointestinal bleeding and the following measurements were obtained: diastolic mean gradient 11 mmHg, peak gradient 16 mmHg, pressure half-time 65 ms, heart rate 114/min. This increased gradient is:
    A. Likely normal
    B. Likely abnormal
    C. Cannot comment

11. The following measurements were obtained in a patient with MR: proximal isovelocity surface area (PISA) radius 1 cm at a Nyquist limit of 50 cm/s, peak MR velocity 5 m/s, and MR signal time velocity integral 100 cm. The regurgitant volume is:
    A. 63 cc/beat
    B. 31 cc/beat
    C. 63 cc/s
    D. 63%

12. Distribution of leaflet thickening and calcification in rheumatic mitral stenosis is:
    A. More at the tip
    B. More at the base
    C. Uniform throughout the leaflets

13. Leaflet calcification in degenerative mitral stenosis is:
    A. More at the tip
    B. More at the base
    C. Uniform throughout the leaflets

14. The predominant mechanism of chronic ischemic MR is:
    A. Restriction of mitral leaflet closure
    B. Papillary muscle dysfunction
    C. Ruptured chordae tendinae
    D. Ruptured papillary muscle

15. In a person with chronic ischemic MR due to old inferior myocardial infarction (MI) and an ejection fraction of 50%, the location of the MR jet would be:
    A. Medial commissure
    B. Lateral commissure
    C. Central

16. In the patient in Question 15, the jet direction would be:
    A. Posterior
    B. Anterior
    C. Central

17. In a patient with old anteroseptal MI with an ejection fraction of 28%, an ischemic MR jet is likely to be:
    A. Central
    B. Lateral wall hugging
    C. Medial wall hugging

18. MR in aortic stenosis is related to which of these factors:
    A. Degree of mitral annular calcification
    B. Severity of aortic stenosis
    C. An increase in left ventricular (LV) end systolic dimension
    D. Degree of aortic leaflet calcification

19. Left atrial myxoma may be differentiated from a left atrial thrombus by all of the following characteristics except:
    A. Enhancement with transpulmonary contrast agent
    B. Presence of blood vessels on color flow imaging
    C. Attachment to the atrial septum
    D. Similar mass in the LV with normal LV function.

20. The most common location of a left atrial thrombus is:
    A. Left atrial appendage
    B. Body
    C. Atrial septum
    D. Atrial roof

Answers for Chapter 7

1. **Answer: B.**
   Bicuspid valve is associated with coarctation of the aorta. Biscuspid aortic valve occurs in 1–2% of the population. In these people aortic coarctation is rare, but 25% of patients with coarctation have a bicuspid aortic valve.

2. **Answer: E.**
   Coronary sinus can be dilated due to increased pressure or flow. There is an increased flow in the coronary sinus in the left superior vena cava, which drains into the coronary sinus, coronary A–V fistula due to increased shunt, and unroofed coronary sinus due to increased flow from the left atrium (LA) to coronary sinus. Right atrial hypertension causes increased pressure, which will lead to dilated coronary sinus.

3. **Answer: A.**
   ASD of sinus venosus type is most commonly associated with anomalous drainage of the right upper pulmonary vein into the right atrium.

4. **Answer: A.**
   Ostium primum ASD is most commonly associated with a cleft anterior mitral leaflet. This is a form of endocardial cushion defect or partial AV canal defect.

5. **Answer: C.**
   Infundibular pulmonary stenosis is not associated with dilatation of the pulmonary artery. Poststenotic dilatation is seen only in valvular pulmonary stenosis and not in subvalvular pulmonary stenosis. In ASD the pulmonary artery dilates due to increased flow and pulmonary hypertension dilatation is due to increased pressure. Idiopathic dilatation of the pulmonary artery can also occur. Marfan syndrome is a cause of pulmonary artery dilatation as well.

6. **Answer: D.**
   All conditions except mitral stenosis have weakened media predisposing to dissection. Hypertension can also increase the risk for dissection. There is aortopathy in Marfan syndrome and bicuspid aortic valve. Progesterone in pregnancy loosens connective tissue and may result in aortic as well as coronary dissection.

7. **Answer: A.**
   Normal IVRT is 70–100 ms, and pressure half-time is 65–80 ms for a prosthetic mitral valve. With a normal cardiac output, the mean gradient would be 3–4 mmHg at a heart rate of 60/min. Shortened IVRT, short pressure half-time, and high E/A ratio indicate high LA pressure. A stenotic prosthetic valve would have caused increase in pressure half-time and an increase in mean gradient far more than 6 mmHg at a heart rate of 60/min. A mildly increased gradient despite a shortened pressure half-time indicates increased transvalvular flow suggestive of MR, which may be difficult to visualize from a transthoracic echo. Hence, a transesophageal echocardiogram (TEE) would be warranted. High LA pressure without an increase in flow would result in shortened IVRT and pressure half-time without an increase in the gradient. A good example of this is superadded restrictive cardiomyopathy.

8. **Answer: A.**
   Shadowing in the left atrium is least with a parasternal long axis view; however, TEE is the best technique to evaluate for paravalvular mitral leaks.

9. **Answer: C.**
An unchanged V_1/V_2 ratio compared to prior echo confirms the absence of prosthetic valve stenosis. An elevated V_1 indicates elevated cardiac output and the transvalvular gradient is flow dependent. Anemia is a common problem secondary to blood loss due to anticoagulation and less commonly due to mechanical hemolysis. Patient–prosthesis mismatch occurs when the valve is too small for the cardiac output needs of the patient. The effective aortic orifice area in this patient is about 1.3 cm². There is no change in the intrinsic valvular function in this patient.

10. **Answer: A.**
The measurements are normal. Pressure half-time of 65 ms indicates normal valve function. Mean gradient is appropriately increased due to tachycardia (which shortens the diastolic filling period), anemia, and possibly high cardiac output. Prosthetic valves are intrinsically mildly stenotic.

11. **Answer: A.**
Effective regurgitant orifice area is given by the formula $2\pi r^2 \times$ Nyquist limit/MR velocity, that is, $2 \times 3.14 \times 1 \times 1 \times 50/500\,cm/s = 0.628\,cm^2$. Regurgitant volume is effective regurgitant orifice area (in cm²) × TVI (in cm). In this patient it is $0.628 \times 100 = 62.8\,cc$. This is per beat and not per second.

12. **Answer: A.**

13. **Answer: B.**
Calcification extends from the annulus, that is, in a centripetal fashion in contrast to rheumatic, which is centrifugal or more at the tip.

14. **Answer: A.**
Restriction, tethering, and tenting refer to the phenomenon of incomplete systolic closure due to apical traction on the mitral leaflets due to outward displacement of the papillary muscles. This causes tenting of the leaflets, and the coaptation point is displaced apically. This is not due to contractile failure of the papillary muscles (papillary muscle dysfunction). Papillary muscle rupture causes acute MR, leading to pulmonary edema and hemodynamic compromise. Tenting is far more common than papillary muscle rupture.

15. **Answer: A.**
Owing to displacement of the posteromedial papillary muscle, there is tethering of the medial portions of both leaflet (P3 and A3) segments causing a medial commissural jet. When the left ventricle (LV) is uniformly dilated, the jet could be central in origin.

16. **Answer: A.**
As there is greater tenting of P3 than A3, the jet is directed posteriorly. There may also be some tenting of P2.

17. **Answer: A.**
In an anterior MI, there is generally remodeling of the noninfarcted segments as well, causing dilatation of the whole LV cavity. This is reflected by a low ejection fraction. This causes displacement of both papillary muscles and tenting of all segments of both leaflets, giving rise to central MR, although exceptions may occur. MR in dilated cardiomyopathy occurs because of a similar mechanism.

18. **Answer: C.**

    The mechanism of MR is functional and is related to LV dilatation and leaflet tethering. Aortic leaflet calcification, mitral annular calcification, and severity of aortic stenosis contribute very little in the genesis of MR. A higher driving pressure in more severe degrees of aortic stenosis may increase the regurgitant volume and the jet area but will not cause MR in the absence of a defect in the mitral coaptation mechanism.

19. **Answer: C.**

    Myxomas are vascular; blood vessels may be seen on color flow imaging and enhanced mildly with transpulmonary contrast agent. Although left atrial thrombus is most commonly seen in the appendage, it may be attached to the atrial septum or may traverse through a patent foramen ovale from the right side (paradoxical embolism). The presence of a mass in the LV in the face of normal LV function makes a thrombus unlikely and points to a familial myxoma syndrome (Carney's syndrome).

20. **Answer: A.**

    This generally occurs in the presence of atrial fibrillation or flutter. The probability is increased by the presence of mitral stenosis, heart failure, low ejection fraction, large left atrium, and left atrial spontaneous echo contrast.

8

Questions

1. The most common benign tumor in the heart is:
   A. Left atrial myxoma
   B. Papillary fibroelastoma
   C. Lambl's excrescences
   D. Fibroma

2. The most common metastatic malignant tumor of the heart is:
   A. Melanoma
   B. Lung cancer
   C. Breast cancer
   D. Renal cancer

3. In a person with flail P2 segment of the posterior mitral leaflet (PML), the mitral regurgitation (MR) jet is likely to be:
   A. Posterior wall hugging
   B. Anterior wall hugging
   C. Central
   D. Cannot comment

4. In a person with flail A2 segment of the anterior mitral leaflet (AML), the MR jet is likely to be:
   A. Posterior wall hugging
   B. Anterior wall hugging
   C. Central
   D. Cannot comment

5. Total surface area of mitral leaflets is generally ____% of mitral annular area:
   A. 100%
   B. 120%
   C. 150%
   D. 200%

Echocardiography Board Review: 600 Multiple Choice Questions with Discussion, Third Edition.
Ramdas G. Pai and Padmini Varadarajan.
© 2025 John Wiley & Sons Ltd. Published 2025 by John Wiley & Sons Ltd.

6. The PML compared to the AML is:
   A. Shorter
   B. Longer
   C. The same length as the anterior leaflet
   D. Of variable length

7. The length of the posterior leaflet attachment to the mitral annulus compared to that of the AML is:
   A. Shorter
   B. Longer
   C. The same
   D. Variable

8. In an apical long axis view the following mitral leaflet segments are seen:
   A. A2P2
   B. A3P3
   C. A1P1
   D. A3P1

9. Apical two-chamber view is likely to show the following mitral leaflet segments:
   A. P1A2P3
   B. A2P2
   C. A3P1
   D. A1P1

10. The major diameter of the mitral annulus is best imaged from:
    A. Apical two-chamber view
    B. Apical long axis view
    C. Apical five-chamber view
    D. Parasternal long axis view

11. The MR jet is best visualized in parasternal long axis view when the transducer tip is directed more inferomedially. The location of the MR jet in this patient is:
    A. Medial commissure
    B. Lateral commissure
    C. Central

12. A continuous flow is visualized in the main pulmonary artery. This could be related to:
    A. Patent ductus arteriosus (PDA)
    B. Coronary A–V fistula
    C. Idiopathic dilatation of main pulmonary artery
    D. None of the above

13. Echocardiographic features of anatomic right ventricle in a congenitally corrected transposition of great vessels are all of the following except:
    A. Trileaflet atrioventricular valve
    B. Apical position of associated atrioventricular valve
    C. Presence of moderator band
    D. Wall thickness < 7 mm

14. Problems encountered with congenitally corrected great arteries are all of the following except:
    A. Failure of systemic ventricle
    B. Tricuspid regurgitation

    C. Atrial and ventricular arrhythmias

    D. Aortic regurgitation

15. Features of tetralogy of Fallot are all of the following except:
    A. Overriding aorta
    B. Nonrestrictive ventricular septal defect (VSD)
    C. Pulmonary stenosis
    D. Right ventricular (RV) hypertrophy
    E. Atrial septal defect (ASD)

16. Associations of atrial septal aneurysm include all of the following except:
    A. Patent foramen ovale
    B. Atrial arrythmias
    C. Transient ischemic attacks
    D. Pulmonary hypertension

17. Echocardiographic findings in Ebstein's anomaly may include:
    A. Apical displacement of the septal leaflet of the tricuspid valve > 8 mm compared to position of anterior mitral leaflet attachment
    B. Large septal tricuspid leaflet with tethering to RV wall
    C. Tricuspid regurgitation
    D. ASD
    E. Hypoplastic pulmonary arteries

18. The most common location of the accessory pathway in Ebstein's anomaly is:
    A. Posteroseptal
    B. Anteroseptal
    C. Right lateral
    D. Left lateral

19. The following type of VSD is likely to be associated with aortic regurgitation:
    A. Perimembranous
    B. Muscular
    C. Supracristal
    D. Inlet

20. In a patient with secundum ASD, the following features are consistent with amenability of percutaneous closure except:
    A. Defect size of 22 mm
    B. Mitral rim of 8 mm
    C. Aortic rim of 2 mm
    D. Inferior vena cava rim of 1 mm

Answers for Chapter 8

1. **Answer: B.**
Papillary fibroelastoma is the most common benign tumor seen in the heart, followed by myxoma. Lambl's excrescences are not tumors; they are fibrinous strands mostly found on the aortic valve.

2. **Answer: B.**
The most common metastatic malignancy of the heart is lung, followed by breast cancer. Melanoma has the potential to metastasize to myocardium but is not the commonest to metastasize to the heart. Primary malignant tumors of the heart are rare, but myxoma followed by rhabdomyoma are the commonest. Of the malignant type, sarcomas are the commonest to affect the heart. Metastatic tumors are about 100 times as common compared with primary malignant tumors of the heart. About 50% of melanomas metastasize. Primary cardiac lymphoma is very rare and is typically of non-Hodgkin's type. It typically only involves the heart and pericardium with very minimal extracardiac involvement. It accounts for only 1% of primary cardiac tumors and 0.5% of the extranodal lymphomas. In immunocompetent hosts it is usually a diffuse B-cell lymphoma and in immunosuppressed hosts small noncleaved or immunoblastic are more common. The right atrium and right ventricle are the two most common sites involved.

3. **Answer: B.**
The jet is away from the flail segment in contrast to a tethered segment.

4. **Answer: A.**

5. **Answer: C.**
Normally there is 50% more leaflet tissue than annular area to cause a 2–3 mm leaflet overlap at the coaptation margin. The absolute leaflet area is increased in myxomatous mitral valve disease and hypertrophic cardiomyopathy. The normal annular area is roughly 7–8 cm^2 and the leaflet area is 10–12 cm^2.

6. **Answer: A.**
The posterior leaflet length is 10–14 mm and the anterior leaflet length is 20–24 mm.

7. **Answer: B.**
This results in equal surface area of anterior and posterior leaflets.

8. **Answer: A.**
This view cuts through the middle of both leaflets, that is, A2 and P2.

9. **Answer: A.**
Two-chamber view goes through the intercommissural plane and cuts through P1 and P3, with A2 seen between them in systole. A medial tilt of the transducer will cut the AML entirely showing A1A2A3, and a lateral tilt will cut the PML entirely revealing P1P2P3.

10. **Answer: A.**
Equivalent to this on a transesophageal echocardiogram (TEE) examination is the mid-esophageal view at 70–80 degrees. Apical long axis view gives the minor dimension of the mitral annulus.

11. **Answer: A.**
Tilting the transducer from this location toward the left shoulder will reveal the lateral commissure.

12. **Answer: A.**
    The PDA drains at the origin of the left pulmonary artery. Anomalous origin of the coronary artery from the pulmonary artery can cause continuous flow because of retrograde flow into the pulmonary artery. Both are examples of left to right shunts. Dilatation of the pulmonary artery can cause swirling of blood in the pulmonary artery in systole, giving a false impression of shunt flow because of reversed flow direction.

13. **Answer: D.**
    Ventricles go with corresponding atrioventricular valves, that is, right ventricle with tricuspid valve that is apically positioned and left ventricle with mitral valve. Wall thickness is not a reliable feature. In right ventricular hypertrophy the wall thickness may be > 7 mm, and the pulmonary left ventricle may have a wall thickness of < 7 mm.

14. **Answer: D.**
    The systemic RV has a high likelihood of failure. It may also have myocardial perfusion defects. Tricuspid valve failure (systemic atrioventricular valve) is common secondary to annular dilatation. Atrial and ventricular arrhythmias are common due to dilatation of the left atrium and systemic RV. Presence of atrial arrhythmias may contribute to RV dysfunction.

15. **Answer: E.**
    ASD is not a feature in classical tetralogy of Fallot. Presence of ASD in tetralogy has been referred to as the pentalogy of Fallot.

16. **Answer: D.**
    The left to right shunt through the patent foramen ovale (PFO) is generally very small and hence pulmonary hypertension is not seen with an aneurysmal atrial septum. Risk of transient ischemic attack is highest when PFO and atrial septal aneurysm coexist and the shunt flow is large. Speculated mechanisms for this include paradoxical embolism, in situ thrombus formation, and atrial arrhythmias.

17. **Answer: E.**
    Hypoplastic pulmonary arteries are not a feature. ASD may coexist and in the presence of tricuspid regurgitation may result in right to left shunt, causing cyanosis.

18. **Answer: C.**
    Right lateral.

19. **Answer: C.**
    In this type of VSD, there is loss of support to the right coronary cusp of the aortic valve, which will result in aortic regurgitation.

20. **Answer: D.**
    The maximum stretched diameter of the defect that can be closed is 40 mm with an Amplatzer device provided that the septum is large enough to allow the 8 mm flange all around, making the total disk diameter on the left atrial side 56 mm. Aortic rim is the least important and not essential. Inadequacy of other rims may result not only in impingement of the disks on related structures but device instability and dislodgment. Proximity of superior vena cava rim to the right upper pulmonary vein is important as well.

CHAPTER 9

9

Questions

1. Diagnostic sensitivity of stress echocardiography is higher with:
   A. One-vessel disease
   B. Two-vessel disease
   C. Three-vessel disease
   D. Sensitivity is not affected by number of vessels involved

2. False-positive rate for stress echocardiography is high in this group of patients:
   A. Low probability of coronary artery disease (CAD)
   B. Intermediate probability of CAD
   C. High probability of CAD
   D. Independent of CAD

3. Negative predictive value of stress echo is lowest in this group of patients:
   A. Low probability of CAD
   B. Intermediate probability of CAD
   C. High probability of CAD
   D. Independent of CAD

4. False-positive wall motion abnormalities are most commonly seen in this myocardial segment:
   A. Posterior basal wall
   B. Anterior septum
   C. Lateral wall
   D. Apex

5. The most common normal response of left ventricular (LV) end systolic size during exercise is:
   A. Reduction
   B. Increase
   C. Variable response
   D. No change

Echocardiography Board Review: 600 Multiple Choice Questions with Discussion, Third Edition.
Ramdas G. Pai and Padmini Varadarajan.
© 2025 John Wiley & Sons Ltd. Published 2025 by John Wiley & Sons Ltd.

6. An increase in LV end systolic volume during stress may occur in all of these situations except:
   A. Multivessel CAD
   B. Left main CAD
   C. Hypertensive blood pressure response
   D. Left ventricular hypertrophy

7. A 53-year-old patient is undergoing dobutamine stress echocardiography (DSE). At 20 µg dose, the blood pressure drops from 140/80 mmHg to 80/50 mmHg associated with severe nausea, and the heart rate drops from 110/min to 60/min. The most likely cause of this response is:
   A. Left ventricular cavity obliteration causing a vagal response
   B. Severe ischemic response due to multivessel CAD
   C. 2:1 A–V block produced by ischemia in right coronary artery territory
   D. None of the above

8. This proportion of normal patients undergoing DSE may have a drop in their blood pressure:
   A. Zero
   B. 20%
   C. 50%
   D. 89%

9. All of the following factors affect pulmonary vein A-wave amplitude except:
   A. LV end diastolic stiffness
   B. Left atrial function
   C. Pulmonary vein diameter
   D. Heart rate
   E. Pulmonary artery pressure

10. The pulmonary vein S-wave may be less prominent than the D-wave in the following situations except:
    A. Young children
    B. Moderate to severe mitral regurgitation
    C. Atrial fibrillation
    D. Elevated left atrial (LA) pressure
    E. Abnormal LV relaxation with normal LA pressure

11. Normal pulmonary vein A-wave duration compared with mitral A-wave duration is:
    A. Less
    B. More
    C. The same
    D. Variable

12. Normal pulmonary vein D-wave deceleration in an adult is:
    A. 50–100 ms
    B. 100–170 ms
    C. 170–260 ms
    D. Highly variable

13. Increased pulmonary vein D-wave deceleration time may be encountered in:
    A. Mitral stenosis
    B. Mitral regurgitation

C. High LA pressure

D. Pulmonary valve stenosis

14. Normal mitral E-wave propagation velocity by color M mode inside the LV is:
    A. 10–30 cm/s
    B. 30–50 cm/s
    C. Greater than 50 cm/s
    D. Greater than 500 cm/s

15. A reduced mitral E-wave propagation velocity indicates:
    A. High LA pressure
    B. Increased tau
    C. Reduced tau
    D. Increased modulus LV chamber stiffness

16. A reduced A-wave transit time to the LV outflow tract is indicative of:
    A. Low negative dp/dt
    B. Increased tau
    C. Reduced tau
    D. Increased modulus of LV chamber stiffness

17. Rate of acceleration of the early portion of the aortic regurgitation (AR) signal is determined by:
    A. LV negative dp/dt
    B. LV positive dp/dt
    C. LV end diastolic pressure
    D. Aortic end diastolic pressure

18. Rapidly decelerating terminal portion of the AR signal is mainly influenced by:
    A. LV negative dp/dt
    B. LV positive dp/dt
    C. LV end diastolic pressure
    D. Aortic end diastolic pressure

19. A patient has mild mitral regurgitation and the time taken for mitral regurgitation velocity to drop from 3 m/s velocity to 1 m/s on continuous wave Doppler examination was 40 ms. The average rate of LV pressure decay in this patient is:
    A. 3600 mmHg/s
    B. 1280 mm/s
    C. 800 mm/s
    D. 400 mm/s

20. By tissue velocity imaging, the mitral annular Sm wave is produced by:
    A. Annular descent during systole
    B. Annular ascent during systole
    C. Atrial contraction
    D. LV relaxation

Answers for Chapter 9

1. **Answer: C.**
   It is about 50% for one-vessel disease and 80% for three-vessel disease.

2. **Answer: A.**
   On the basis of Baye's theorem, the diagnostic accuracy is highest for intermediate probability, and in patients with extremely low probability most of the tests will be false positive, yielding a low positive predictive value (PPV). PPV is the proportion of patients with positive tests who truly have disease. In other words, PPV = TP/(TP+FP).

3. **Answer: C.**
   Testing this group of patients is likely to yield a high proportion of patients with a false-negative test, hence lowering the negative predictive value (NPV). In other words, NPV = TN/TN+FN.

4. **Answer: A.**
   Wall motion abnormality in the posterior basal wall is most difficult to analyze due to a range of normalcy, proximity to valvular plane, and the apical displacement of the wall during systole, which results in imaging of different parts of the inferior wall during systole and diastole in the short axis view. False positivity during stress echocardiography is in the range of 40–50% for this wall.

5. **Answer: A.**
   Reduction due to a combination of reduced systemic vascular resistance (SVR) and increased LV contractility. In some women, left ventricular end systolic volume may not diminish with stress and this is normal.

6. **Answer: D.**
   This is the equivalent of transient ischemic dilatation of the LV on stress nuclear perfusion imaging.

7. **Answer: A.**
   This is typical of a vasovagal response that is preceded by a hyperdynamic response, which triggers this. It may be exaggerated by volume depletion and may potentially be prevented by volume loading. When a hyperdynamic response with cavity obliteration is seen, instead of increasing the dobutamine dose, atropine should be administered to increase the heart rate. This will help to avert a vagal response. Drop in SVR is universal during DSE and may not be fully compensated by cardiac output increase. Systolic anterior movement of anterior mitral leaflet can occur during DSE, especially in patients with LV hypotension who develop a hyperdynamic response, but LV outflow tract obstruction is rarely responsible for hypotension. Hypotension in such patients, when it occurs, is generally due to a vagal response produced by the hyperdynamic LV stimulating the vagal C type of fibers in the LV wall.

8. **Answer: B.**
   Drop in blood pressure during DSE does not have the same clinical significance as in a regular exercise stress test. This is because normal cardiac output increase during DSE is only 50–80%, which is far less than exercise. Dobutamine causes peripheral vasodilatation.

9. **Answer: E.**
   The pulmonary vein A-wave amplitude is increased in the presence of a stiff LV and reduced in left atrial mechanical failure. The pulmonary A-wave may disappear with heart rates in excess of 100/min, where flow may be entirely antegrade, and atrial contraction may produce a transient deceleration pulmonary flow without reversal. As velocity depends upon flow volume and cross-sectional area, a dilated pulmonary vein is likely to reduce the A-wave velocity, and a collapsed vein in a dry patient can result in a giant A-wave.

10. **Answer: E.**
    Young children have very efficient LV relaxation properties, resulting in rapid early filling (mitral E-wave) paralleled by an increase in D-wave that might have rapid deceleration as well. As S1 is due to atrial relaxation, atrial fibrillation results in reduced S-wave amplitude. Systolic left atrial filling from mitral regurgitation will impede pulmonary vein flow in systole. High LA pressure renders the LA less compliant due to rightward shift of its pressure–volume curve and hence will impede atrial systolic filling, as LA is a closed chamber receiving only pulmonary venous flow during systole. Abnormal LV relaxation reduces E- and D-wave amplitudes, resulting in an increase in S-wave amplitude in the absence of elevated LA pressure.

11. **Answer: A.**
    Increased pulmonary A-wave duration compared with mitral A-wave duration indicates high LV end diastolic pressure. Delta duration of more than 30 ms is very suggestive of high LV end diastolic pressure.

12. **Answer: C.**
    Reduced D-wave deceleration time indicates high LA pressure very similar to mitral E-wave deceleration time.

13. **Answer: A.**
    The D-wave deceleration time parallels mitral E-wave deceleration time, and the slope is flatter in mitral stenosis. It may also be prolonged in patients with prosthetic mitral valves and abnormal LV relaxation. The deceleration time is reduced with high left atrial pressure. Pulmonary valve stenosis has no known effect on this slope.

14. **Answer: C.**
    Greater than 50 cm/s. It gets slower with impaired LV relaxation.

15. **Answer: B.**
    Slower propagation indicates abnormal LV relaxation, and this is reflected by increased tau by invasive measurement. Modulus of chamber stiffness is a measure of LV diastolic stiffness, which comes into play in late diastole.

16. **Answer: D.**
    The A-wave propagation is an end diastolic phenomenon and its propagation velocity is increased with increased LV end diastolic stiffness. Increased propagation velocity results in a shorter transit time. The modulus of chamber stiffness is a measure of operative LV stiffness.

17. **Answer: A.**
    Assuming a constant aortic pressure during this short time, rate of acceleration is principally determined by LV pressure decay after aortic valve closure during the LV isovolumic relaxation period. For example, at the 1 m/s point the aortic–LV

pressure gradient is 4 mmHg and at 2.5 m/s it is 25 mmHg. Assuming a constant aortic pressure, the drop in LV pressure between these two points is $25 - 4 = 21$ mmHg. The rate of LV pressure drop would be 21/time taken for AR signal to increase from 1 m/s to 2.5 m/s. For example, if this time interval is 20 ms (0.02 s), the average negative LV dp/dt would be $21/0.02 = 1050$ mmHg/s.

18. **Answer: B.**

    This rapidly decelerating terminal portion of AR occurs during the isovolumic contraction period and the LV positive dp/dt may be calculated with similar assumptions as for the LV negative dp/dt between 2.5 m/s and 1 m/s points of the AR signal.

19. **Answer: C.**

    The LV negative $dp/dt = 36 - 4/0.04 = 800$ mmHg/s. This again assumes a constant LA pressure during this portion of LV isovolumic contraction time. This noninvasive measure has been validated against invasively derived negative dp/dt by high-fidelity LV pressure recordings.

20. **Answer: A.**

    Annular descent produced by LV long axis shortening causes a positive systolic deflection recorded from the apical view.

10

Questions

1. In a normal heart, compared to timing of mitral E-wave peak, mitral annular Em peak is:
   A. Earlier
   B. Later
   C. Simultaneous
   D. No relationship

2. Post-ejection left ventricular (LV) shortening may be found in all of the following conditions except:
   A. Hypertensive heart disease
   B. Ischemic cardiomyopathy
   C. Cardiac syndrome X
   D. Mitral stenosis

3. Compared to the epicardial, endocardial radial velocities are:
   A. Higher
   B. Lower
   C. Similar
   D. Variable

4. The following myocardial velocities were obtained from the posterior wall by color Doppler tissue imaging: peak systolic epicardial velocity 2 cm/s, peak systolic endocardial velocity 16 cm/s, systolic LV wall thickness 1.4 cm, early diastolic epicardial velocity 3 cm/s, endocardial velocity 18 cm/s, and diastolic wall thickness 1 cm. The systolic transmural velocity gradient in this patient is:
   A. 10/s
   B. 14 cm/s
   C. 19.6 cm/s
   D. 19.6/s

Echocardiography Board Review: 600 Multiple Choice Questions with Discussion, Third Edition.
Ramdas G. Pai and Padmini Varadarajan.
© 2025 John Wiley & Sons Ltd. Published 2025 by John Wiley & Sons Ltd.

5. For the patient in Question 4, diastolic myocardial velocity gradient for the posterior wall is:
   A. 15/s
   B. 1.5/s
   C. 18/s
   D. 18 cm/s

6. In a person with cardiomyopathy, the following Doppler measurements were obtained: Q wave to aortic flow 140 ms, Q wave to pulmonary flow 70 ms, Q to medial mitral annular Sm wave 70 ms, Q to anterior mitral annular Sm wave 85 ms, Q to lateral Sm wave 140 ms, and Q to posterior wall Sm wave 130 ms. *Interventricular* asynchrony in this patient is:
   A. 70 ms
   B. 140 ms
   C. 85 ms
   D. 50 ms

7. In the patient in Question 6, LV *intraventricular* asynchrony is:
   A. 70 ms
   B. 140 ms
   C. 85 ms
   D. 130 ms

8. Stroke risk in a patient with patent foramen ovale (PFO) is influenced by:
   A. Size of PFO
   B. Atrial septal aneurysm
   C. History of prior stroke or transient ischemic attack
   D. All of the above
   E. None of the above

9. Atrial septal aneurysm may be associated with:
   A. PFO
   B. Atrial arrythmias
   C. Increased stroke risk
   D. All of the above
   E. None of the above

10. Observational data on percutaneous PFO closure indicate that the benefit is greater with:
    A. Larger PFO
    B. Complete PFO closure
    C. Higher number of previous strokes
    D. All of the above
    E. None of the above

11. All of the following are probable causes of mitral stenosis except:
    A. Rheumatic fever
    B. Excessive calcification of the mitral annulus
    C. Phen-fen valvulopathy
    D. Ischemic heart disease

12. Bicuspid aortic valve (BAV) may be associated with all of the following except:
    A. Aortic root disease
    B. Coarctation of the aorta

C. Aortic stenosis or regurgitation

D. Ventricular septal defect (VSD)

13. The most common cause of aortic stenosis in a 50-year-old individual is:
    A. Calcific
    B. BAV
    C. Unicuspid aortic valve
    D. Rheumatic heart disease

14. Heart failure with normal ejection fraction can occur in the following except:
    A. Hypertrophic cardiomyopathy
    B. Cardiac amyloid
    C. Restrictive cardiomyopathy
    D. Dilated cardiomyopathy

15. The basic components of a partial atrioventricular canal defect include all except:
    A. Inlet VSD
    B. Septum primum atrial septal defect
    C. Cleft mitral valve
    D. Widened anteroseptal tricuspid commissure and cleft in septal tricuspid leaflet

16. Signs of acute aortic regurgitation include:
    A. Premature mitral valve closure
    B. Hyperdynamic LV function
    C. Normal LV size
    D. All of the above
    E. None of the above

17. The following are indicative of severe mitral regurgitation except:
    A. Systolic flow reversal in the pulmonary veins
    B. Regurgitant fraction of > 60%
    C. Effective regurgitant orifice area of $\geq 0.4\,cm^2$
    D. Vena contracta diameter of $\geq 3\,mm$

18. The following are signs of chronic severe aortic regurgitation except:
    A. Regurgitant fraction $\geq 60\%$
    B. Regurgitant volume of $\geq 60\,cc$
    C. Effective regurgitation orifice area $\geq 0.2\,cm^2$
    D. Vena contracta width $\geq 0.6\,cm$

19. Prosthetic valve gradients are increased in the following conditions except:
    A. Anemia
    B. Febrile state
    C. LV diastolic dysfunction
    D. Hyperthyroidism

20. What is the velocity of circumferential fiber shortening (VCF) in a patient with the following measurements: LV end diastolic dimension 50 mm, end systolic dimension 33 mm, LV ejection time 300 ms.
    A. 1.1
    B. 0.9
    C. 34
    D. Cannot be calculated

Answers for Chapter 10

1. **Answer: A.**
   The Em peak precedes the mitral E peak in normals. This early LV lengthening is due to a combination of LV recoil and relaxation, which generates the mitral E-wave. In patients with abnormal LV relaxation, the Em peak may follow the E-wave peak, the E-wave mainly driven by LA pressure.

2. **Answer: D.**
   Post-ejection LV shortening is the phenomenon of continued myocardial segmental contraction even after the end of ejection. This asynchrony of the ending of LV contraction may result in impaired LV pressure decay or relaxation and hence impaired LV filling. It is found in a variety of disorders affecting the LV.

3. **Answer: A.**
   This results in a myocardial velocity gradient. A transmural myocardial velocity gradient is a better index of contractile function compared to endocardial myocardial velocities alone. The myocardial velocity gradient is obtained as (endocardial velocity – epicardial velocity)/LV wall thickness and reflects the rate of LV wall thickening.

4. **Answer: A.**
   Systolic myocardial velocity gradient = $(16 - 2\,cm/s)/1.4\,cm = 10/s$.

5. **Answer: A.**
   Diastolic myocardial velocity gradient = $(18 - 3\,cm/s)/1\,cm = 15/s$.

6. **Answer: A.**
   Interventricular asynchrony is the difference between the time difference in the onset of mechanical systolies of right and left ventricles, generally measured as the time difference in right ventricular (RV) and LV ejection from the corresponding flows at pulmonary and aortic valves. In this patient, the electromechanical delay for the RV was 70 ms and for the LV was 140 ms. The difference is 70 ms, which corresponds to *interventricular* asynchrony or dyssynchrony.

7. **Answer: A.**
   The largest difference between electromechanical delays in the LV is a measure of intraventricular mechanical asynchrony. In this patient $140 - 70 = 70$ ms corresponds to *intraventricular* asynchrony (LV septolateral delay). Greater than 65 ms is a good predictor for response in terms of reverse remodeling and symptom improvement. As the peak velocities are easier to identify, most of the investigators currently use time to peak velocity rather than time to onset.

8. **Answer: D.**
   Risk of stroke is higher in those with a large PFO, associated with an aneurysmal fossa ovalis, large right to left shunt on saline contrast, and prior embolic events.

9. **Answer: D.**

10. **Answer: D.**
    Randomized trials have to some extent supported observational data. The CLOSE and REDUCE trials showed a benefit of PFO closure with antiplatelet therapy in patients with cryptogenic stroke and large PFOs with right to left

shunts (both NEJM 2017). The NOMAS (Di Tuillo et al., J Am Coll Cardiol. 2007;49(7):797–802) and SPARC (Meissner et al., J Am Coll Cardiol. 2006; 47(2):440–5) studies, which looked at the occurrence of first stroke in patients, found a modest but statistically insignificant association between the baseline presence of PFO and first stroke on follow-up; odds ratio (OR): 1.64 (95% confidence interval (CI) 0.87–3.09) and 1.46 (95% CI 0.74–2.88), respectively. Interestingly, both studies found increased risk of stroke in patients with atrial septal aneurysm alone in the absence of a demonstrable PFO. A meta-analysis of four studies comparing recurrent stroke risk in PFO vs. non-PFO comparison group failed to show an association with a pooled relative risk of 1.1 (95% CI 0.8–1.5) (Almekhlafi et al., Neurology. 2009;73(2):89–97). A more recent study that included 468 patients with cryptogenic stroke showed no difference in recurrent stroke rates in patients with or without PFO or atrial septal aneurysm (Serena et al., Stroke. 2008;39(12):3131–6). PFO closure is not recommended in asymptomatic individuals, to prevent migraine, or in those with deep vein thrombosis and PFO, per Society for Cardiovascular Angiography & Interventions (SCAI) guidelines. But it is indicated in those PFO patients doing deep sea diving and in platypnea-orthodeoxia syndrome.

11. **Answer: D.**
Ischemic heart disease causes mitral regurgitation but is not a cause of mitral stenosis. All the others can cause mitral stenosis.

12. **Answer: D.**
VSD does not occur as an association with BAV. Bicuspid aortic disease is autosomal dominant with incomplete penetrance and variable expressivity. There are two main theories to explain the aortopathy: (1) hemodynamic theory and (2) genetic theory. The most BAV form involving fusion of right and left cusps has been linked to aortic root enlargement and asymmetric pattern of dilatation of the ascending aorta. Fusion of right and noncoronary cusps leads to ascending aortic dilatation often up to the transverse arch without root involvement.

13. **Answer: B.**
The most common cause of aortic stenosis in a 50-year-old individual is BAV. Calcific aortic stenosis occurs in individuals older than 70 years. Unicuspid aortic valve occurs in infancy. Rheumatic heart disease occurs in children aged 5–15 years, mostly in developing countries.

14. **Answer: D.**
Dilated cardiomyopathy is associated with systolic heart failure. All the others are associated with heart failure and a normal ejection fraction, due to abnormal diastolic mechanics.

15. **Answer: A.**
When inlet VSD is present along with the other defects, it constitutes complete AV canal defect. Without the presence of inlet VSD, the other three findings constitute a partial AV canal defect. In partial AV canal defect, mitral and tricuspid annuli are separate.

16. **Answer: D.**
In acute AR, there is no LV dilatation. Hence, in acute AR an increase in LV end diastolic pressure results in premature closure of the mitral valve.

17. **Answer: D.**
    A vena contracta width of $\geq 0.7\,cm$ is suggestive of severe MR. The rest of the choices are indicative of severe MR.

18. **Answer: C.**
    Effective orifice area in chronic severe aortic regurgitation is $\geq 0.3\,cm^2$. All the other findings are suggestive of severe aortic regurgitation.

19. **Answer: C.**
    All the other states except LV diastolic dysfunction can cause an increase in prosthetic valve gradients due to increased stroke volume.

20. **Answer: A.**
    VCF = fractional shortening/ejection time in seconds. Fractional shortening is a measure of degree of shortening of endocardial circumference. In this patient, fractional shortening = $(50-33)/50 = 0.34$. Thus, VCF is $0.34/0.3 = 1.1$ circumferences/s.

11

Questions

1. Principal determinants of left ventricular (LV) end systolic circumferential wall stress include all of the following except:
   A. LV end systolic dimension
   B. LV end systolic pressure
   C. LV systolic wall thickness
   D. LV pressure at mitral valve closure

2. Increase in LV end systolic wall stress is likely to reduce all of the following except:
   A. Ejection fraction
   B. Fractional shortening
   C. Velocity of circumferential shortening
   D. LV positive dp/dt

3. The response of LV end systolic volume to an increase in LV end systolic wall stress would be:
   A. An increase
   B. A decrease
   C. No change

4. In a person with LV dysfunction, compared to a normal individual, a graph showing end systolic wall stress (ESWS) on the x-axis and end systolic volume (ESV) on the y-axis would be:
   A. Steeper
   B. Flatter
   C. None of the above

5. In response to dobutamine infusion, the ESV–ESWS curve will shift:
   A. Downward
   B. Upward
   C. No shift

Echocardiography Board Review: 600 Multiple Choice Questions with Discussion, Third Edition.
Ramdas G. Pai and Padmini Varadarajan.
© 2025 John Wiley & Sons Ltd. Published 2025 by John Wiley & Sons Ltd.

6. The factor least likely to affect the mitral E/A ratio is:
   A. Tau
   B. Modulus of LV chamber stiffness
   C. Left atrial pressure
   D. LV elastic recoil
   E. Cardioversion for atrial fibrillation performed 2 hours ago
   F. Pulmonary artery pressure

7. Factors affecting LV isovolumic relaxation time (IVRT) are all of the following except:
   A. Tau
   B. Left atrial pressure
   C. Heart rate
   D. Moderate aortic regurgitation

8. The factor least likely to diminish mitral A-wave amplitude is:
   A. Recent cardioversion
   B. Myopathic left atrium
   C. An acute rise in LV end diastolic pressure (LVEDP)
   D. Severe aortic stenosis with mild LV hypertrophy and normal LV ejection fraction

9. Both high left atrial (LA) pressure and atrial mechanical failure result in a high E/A ratio. The following is least likely to help in the differential diagnosis in this situation:
   A. E-wave deceleration time
   B. Amplitude and duration of AR-wave
   C. Pulmonary vein S/D time velocity integral ratio
   D. Mitral annular velocity with tissue Doppler imaging

10. This change is least likely to occur in a patient with acute severe aortic regurgitation:
    A. Reduction of A-wave amplitude
    B. Premature presystolic closure of the mitral valve
    C. Diastolic mitral regurgitation
    D. Increased amplitude and duration of pulmonary AR-wave
    E. A decrease in mitral Em-wave amplitude

11. A late peaking systolic velocity signal is found in the following condition:
    A. Mitral valve prolapse causing late systolic mitral regurgitation (MR)
    B. MR due to systolic anterior motion of the mitral leaflet
    C. LV cavity obliteration
    D. Acute severe MR

12. The following condition causes a reduction in the acceleration time of pulmonary arterial flow:
    A. Pulmonary stenosis
    B. Pulmonary hypertension
    C. Dilated pulmonary artery
    D. Right ventricular (RV) dysfunction

13. Increased respirophasic variations in transvalvular flows may occur in all of the following conditions except:
    A. Status asthmaticus
    B. Constrictive pericarditis

C. Cardiac tamponade

D. A large RV infarct

E. Hypovolemic shock

14. Intrapericardial pressure is increased in all of the following conditions except:
    A. Cardiac tamponade
    B. Acute massive pulmonary embolism
    C. Acute traumatic rupture of tricuspid valve, causing acute tricuspid regurgitation
    D. Acute RV infarct
    E. Severe aortic stenosis with normal LV function

15. A patient with a St. Jude mitral valve no. 29 has a mean diastolic gradient of 3 mmHg and a pressure half-time of 70 ms at a heart rate of 70 beats/min. This is consistent with:
    A. Normal prosthetic valve function
    B. Prosthetic valve thrombosis
    C. Significant pannus growth
    D. Severe MR

16. A patient with a St. Jude mitral prosthetic valve no. 29 has a mean diastolic gradient of 7 mmHg at a heart rate of 70 beats/min and a pressure half-time of 30 ms. This is consistent with:
    A. Normal prosthetic valve function
    B. Prosthetic valve thrombosis
    C. Significant pannus growth
    D. Severe MR

17. A patient with a prosthetic mitral valve no. 29 has a mean diastolic gradient of 10 mmHg at a heart rate of 70 beats/min and a pressure half-time of 200 ms. This is consistent with:
    A. Normal prosthetic valve function
    B. Prosthetic mitral valve stenosis
    C. Severe anemia with high output failure
    D. Severe MR

18. The A2–OS snap interval corresponds to:
    A. Isovolumic relaxation time
    B. Isovolumic contraction time
    C. Pre-ejection period
    D. All of the above

19. In a patient with mitral valve stenosis, the A2–OS interval may be shortened by all of the following except:
    A. Severe mitral stenosis
    B. Severe MR
    C. Tachycardia
    D. Abnormal LV relaxation

20. An abnormal LV relaxation pattern is consistent with:
    A. Mean LA pressure of 10 mmHg and LVEDP of 22 mmHg
    B. Mean LA pressure of 22 mmHg and LVEDP of 10 mmHg
    C. Mean LA pressure of 10 mmHg and LVEDP of 12 mmHg
    D. Mean LA pressure of 28 mmHg and LVEDP of 30 mmHg
    E. Mean LA pressure of 28 mmHg and LVEDP of 40 mmHg

Answers for Chapter 11

1. **Answer: D.**
Systolic wall stress is the force that myocardial fibers have to overcome in order to affect circumferential shortening. It is proportional to LV size and intracavity pressure and inversely proportional to wall thickness. There are three types of wall stresses operating on the myocardium: circumferential, radial, and meridional.

2. **Answer: D.**
The first three measures are afterload dependent and positive dp/dt is preload dependent. LV ESWS is a good measure of afterload, whereas LV end diastolic wall stress is a good measure of preload.

3. **Answer: A.**
An increase. ESWS/ESV is a good load-independent measure of LV systolic performance; a decrease suggests reduced performance, as this indicates a larger ESV for a given ESWS.

4. **Answer: A.**
An increment in ESV in response to an increase in ESWS is greater in a person with LV dysfunction, making this relationship steeper. Contractile responses to changes in afterload may also be studied by using ejection fraction or fractional shortening in place of ESV. However, the response will be in the opposite direction. Also, noninvasively derived LV end systolic pressure (from cuff pressure and carotid pulse tracing) is a reasonable surrogate for ESWS.

5. **Answer: A.**
Dobutamine brings out the LV contractile reserve, causing a reduction in LV end systolic volume for a given ESWS.

6. **Answer: F.**
Tau is an invasive measure of LV relaxation, impairment of which will reduce the E/A ratio. Modulus of LV chamber stiffness is a measure of LV late diastolic stiffness. This affects the A-wave amplitude. High LA pressure increases the E-wave amplitude. Increased elastic recoil as it occurs in a hypercontractile state increases the E-wave amplitude through a suction effect. Atrial mechanical failure is common after cardioversion for atrial fibrillation and may take 1–20 days for full recovery.

7. **Answer: D.**
Impaired relaxation prolongs IVRT through slowing the LV pressure decay between aortic valve closure and mitral valve opening. High LA pressure and a large left atrial V-wave will result in earlier opening of the mitral valve at a higher pressure. Fast heart rate diminishes IVRT partly through an improvement of LV relaxation.

8. **Answer: D.**
Myopathic atrium and recent cardioversion result in reduced A-wave amplitude due to reduced atrial mechanical function. Acute rise in LVEDP results in an acute increase in atrial afterload, diminishing its ejection function, just like any other pumping chamber. Atrial output during its contraction depends upon its preload, afterload, and contractility. In aortic stenosis with LV hypertrophy due to abnormal relaxation, there is reduced early LV filling and a compensatory increase in contribution from left atrial contraction.

9. **Answer: C.**

   High LA pressure results in short IVRT, reduced E-wave deceleration time, and an increase in pulmonary vein AR-wave duration and amplitude. Mitral E/mitral annular Em ratio is a good indicator of LA pressure. Atrial mechanical failure results in diminution of pulmonary AR reversal and absence of atrial relaxation, which causes a left atrial suction effect and will result in diminution of S-wave amplitude. The S-wave amplitude is diminished in high LA pressure due to increased LA operating stiffness during LV systole, when there is no LA emptying.

10. **Answer: E.**

    Acute atrial regurgitation causes a rapid increase in LVEDP, diminishing A-wave amplitude, or eliminating it due to acutely increased atrial afterload. This may also prematurely close the mitral valve. Atrial contraction on a closed mitral valve will result in exaggerated flow reversal in the pulmonary vein during atrial contraction. None of these phenomena directly affects early diastolic LV mechanics, LV relaxation, or early diastolic LV lengthening (Em-wave).

11. **Answer: C.**

    It causes flow acceleration in late systole due to a severe reduction in flow area that occurs in end systole. Although in mitral valve prolapse and hypertrophic obstructive cardiomyopathy the regurgitant volume may be more toward end systole, the shape of the signal is dictated only by the LV–LA pressure gradient and not by the volume of MR. The LV–LA pressure gradient tends to be maximum in early to mid systole. In acute severe MR, a large V-wave causes late systolic deceleration of the signal, a so-called "V-wave cutoff sign."

12. **Answer: B.**

    This is thought to be due to faster return of the reflected pressure waves because of increased operative stiffness of the pulmonary arterial tree, which causes early deceleration of the flow.

13. **Answer: E.**

    In status asthmaticus, exaggerated respiratory variation in intrapleural pressures causes marked variation in venous returns to both the right and left heart during the respiratory cycle. In constriction and tamponade, there is exaggerated interventricular interaction due to septal shifts during respiration, causing an exaggeration of normal flow variations across the valves during the respiratory cycle. RV infarct causes acute RV dilatation and invokes pericardial constraint and physiology similar to constrictive pericarditis.

14. **Answer: E.**

    In addition to pericardial fluid accumulation, any phenomenon that acutely increases the intrapericardial volume invokes pericardial constraint and hence elevation of the intrapericardial pressure. Massive pulmonary embolus and RV infarct cause acute RV dilatation. Any acute regurgitant lesion causes acute chamber dilatation and hence invokes pericardial constraint. Intrapericardial pressure also increases when intrapleural pressure is increased, as in positive end expiratory pressure (PEEP) and tension pneumothorax.

15. **Answer: A.**

    Both the mean gradient and pressure half-time are useful in assessing and monitoring prosthetic mitral valve function.

16. **Answer: D.**
    Reduced pressure half-time is suggestive of high LA pressure, and an increased gradient at a normal heart rate is suggestive of an increased flow across the mitral valve; this combination is highly suggestive of mitral regurgitation.

17. **Answer: B.**
    Stenotic prosthetic valve hemodynamics is similar to native mitral valve stenosis. An increase in gradient is accompanied by an increase in pressure half-time, indicating reduced effective orifice area. High output causes an increase in gradient with a normal or reduced pressure half-time depending upon left atrial pressure.

18. **Answer: A.**
    IVRT is the interval between the aortic component of the second heart sound and mitral valve opening.

19. **Answer: D.**
    High left atrial pressure that occurs in mitral stenosis or MR will cause earlier opening of the mitral valve, thus causing a shortening of the A2–OS interval. Tachycardia improves LV relaxation and shortens this interval. Abnormal LV relaxation, by reducing the rate of pressure decay between aortic valve closure and mitral valve opening, would lengthen this interval.

20. **Answer: A.**
    Abnormal relaxation generally has normal LA pressure but an elevated LVEDP because of a combination of increased contribution of LV filling during atrial systole and possibly increased LV late diastolic stiffness by the same process that caused abnormal LV relaxation. Very high mean LA pressures result in pseudonormal or restrictive LV filling patterns.

CHAPTER 12

12

Questions

1. Which of the following is a potential complication of aortic valve endocarditis?
   A. Aortic root abscess
   B. Supra-annular mitral regurgitation (MR)
   C. Aneurysm of mitral–aortic intervalvular fibrosa
   D. Aneurysm of anterior mitral leaflet
   E. All of the above

2. The following statements are true about patent foramen ovale except:
   A. Pick-up rate is higher with saline contrast compared to color Doppler imaging
   B. Transesophageal echocardiogram (TEE) is more sensitive than transthoracic echocardiogram
   C. Yield is higher with leg injection compared to arm injection for saline contrast
   D. Present in about 50% of the normal population

3. Saline contrast echocardiography in a patient with cirrhosis of the liver showed appearance of contrast in the left atrium five beats after its appearance in the right atrium. This is suggestive of:
   A. Normal physiology
   B. Hepatopulmonary syndrome
   C. Patent foramen ovale
   D. Portopulmonary syndrome

4. Which type of aortic valve is least likely to be repairable for correction of severe aortic regurgitation?
   A. Failure of leaflet coaptation due to severely dilated ascending aorta with structurally normal leaflets
   B. Bicuspid aortic valve with prolapse of the conjoint cusp
   C. Aortic intramural hematoma with extension to the base of right coronary cusp causing it to prolapse
   D. Rheumatic aortic valve disease

5. TEE was performed intraoperatively following coronary artery bypass grafting (CABG) because of failure to wean from cardiopulmonary bypass. It showed

Echocardiography Board Review: 600 Multiple Choice Questions with Discussion, Third Edition.
Ramdas G. Pai and Padmini Varadarajan.
© 2025 John Wiley & Sons Ltd. Published 2025 by John Wiley & Sons Ltd.

akinetic inferior wall with 3+ MR originating at the medial commissure. These findings were not present preoperatively. The inferior wall looked excessively bright. The most likely problem in this patient is:

A. Air embolism into the right coronary artery (RCA)
B. Thrombosis of RCA graft
C. Excessively high blood pressure
D. Excessive intravascular volume
E. Poor myocardial preservation

6. The image is suggestive of:

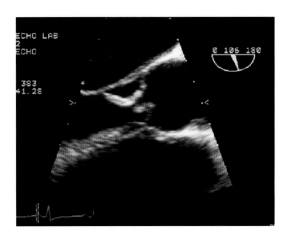

A. Aortic dissection
B. Aortic valve endocarditis
C. Unicuspid aortic valve
D. Hypertrophic cardiomyopathy

7. Continuous wave Doppler shown here could be a result of:

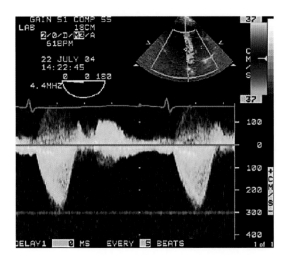

A. Hypertrophic obstructive cardiomyopathy
B. Severe MR
C. Tricuspid regurgitation (TR)
D. Ventricular septal defect

8. In this image, the number 1 denotes:

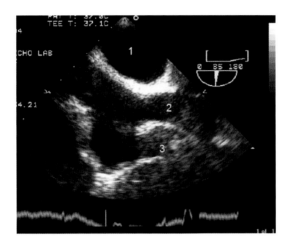

A. Left atrium
B. Right atrium
C. Aorta
D. Right pulmonary artery

9. In this image, the number 2 denotes:

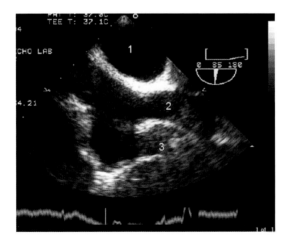

A. Superior vena cava
B. Inferior vena cava
C. Pulmonary artery
D. Aorta

10. In this image, the number 3 denotes:

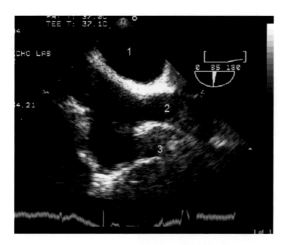

    A. Left atrium
    B. Right atrial appendage
    C. Inferior vena cava
    D. None of the above

11. This image shows:

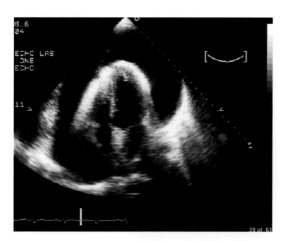

    A. Large left pleural effusion
    B. Large pericardial effusion with no evidence of tamponade
    C. Large pericardial effusion with features of tamponade
    D. Mirror image artifact

12. This mitral inflow pattern is consistent with:

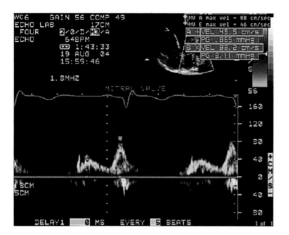

   A. Abnormal left ventricular (LV) relaxation with elevated left atrial (LA) pressure

   B. Abnormal LV relaxation with normal LA pressure

   C. Pseudonormal filling

   D. Restrictive LV filling

13. The part of the flow curve denoted by the arrow in this pulmonary vein flow is caused by:

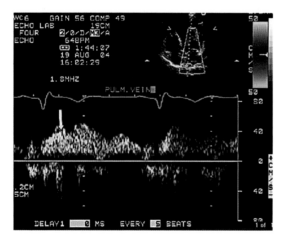

   A. LA relaxation

   B. Right ventricular (RV) ejection

   C. Mitral valve opening

   D. Mitral annular descent

14. The patient shown here has:

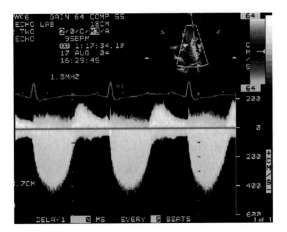

   A. Severe MR
   B. Severe mitral stenosis
   C. Severe aortic stenosis
   D. Mild MR

15. The mitral inflow pattern is consistent with:

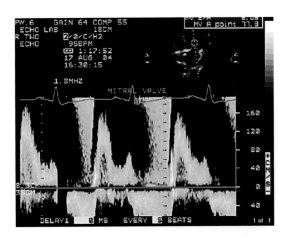

   A. Severe MR
   B. Severe mitral stenosis
   C. Prosthetic mitral valve
   D. Atrial fibrillation

16. In the image shown here, the arrow denotes:

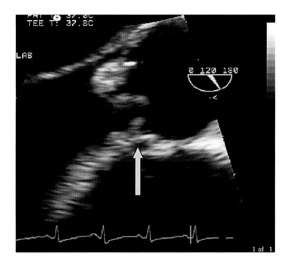

    A. RCA

    B. Coronary sinus

    C. Aortic ring abscess

    D. Prosthetic valve dehiscence

17. The aortic valve shown here is:

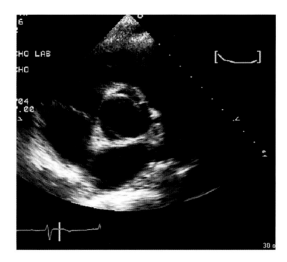

    A. Tricuspid

    B. Unicuspid

    C. Bicuspid with conjoint right and left cusp

    D. Bicuspid with conjoint left and noncoronary cusps

18. This TEE image shows:

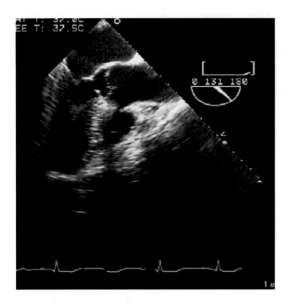

    A. Subaortic membrane
    B. Vegetation
    C. Artifact
    D. Aortic aneurysm

19. This Doppler signal is indicative of:

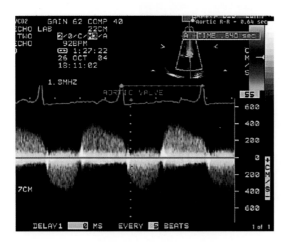

    A. Significant mixed aortic valve disease
    B. Significant mixed mitral valve disease
    C. Significant mixed tricuspid valve disease
    D. Hypertrophic obstructive cardiomyopathy

20. For the patient in Question 19 the LV end diastolic pressure is likely to be:
    A. Low
    B. Normal
    C. Elevated
    D. Cannot comment

Answers for Chapter 12

1. **Answer: E.**
   All of the above. In addition, patients may get aorto-LV fistula, aorto-RV fistula, aorto-RA fistula, anterior mitral leaflet perforation, rupture of the mitral–aortic intervalvular fibrosa, atrioventricular blocks, pyogenic pericarditis, etc.

2. **Answer: D.**
   It is present in about 25% of the normal population. Detection rate is higher with TEE and saline injection especially from the leg, which simulates the direction of flow during fetal life.

3. **Answer: B.**
   Owing to the formation of pulmonary A–V fistulae (caused by "hepatic factor"). This is called hepatopulmonary syndrome. Portopulmonary syndrome refers to pulmonary hypertension secondary to chronic liver disorders. Late appearance of bubbles in the left atrium is indicative of transpulmonary rather than interatrial shunting.

4. **Answer: D.**
   For valve sparing surgery, leaflets should be structurally near normal. In situation A, replacement of ascending aorta may eliminate AR, and in situation C, prolapsing leaflets can be resuspended during repair.

5. **Answer: A.**
   Akinetic wall signifies ischemia, and brightness indicates air embolism into the RCA, the common artery to be affected because of its anterior origin from the aorta. Poor myocardial preservation would cause global hypokinesis. MR in this patient is typically ischemic because of inferior wall motion abnormality.

6. **Answer: B.**
   Large vegetations are seen on the aortic valve. The ascending aorta is normal sized with no visible flap. Unicuspid aortic valve can be diagnosed only in the short axis view showing only a single cusp and a single commissure. In this example, there is a large vegetation on the noncoronary cusp and a smaller one on the right coronary cusp.

7. **Answer: A.**
   Late peaking systolic signal is indicative of dynamic LV outflow tract obstruction, which is most severe in end systole when the LV volume is minimal. The timing corresponds to LV ejection and begins following a period after the onset of the QRS signal. There is a gap between the end of the signal and the onset of mitral inflow. The MR signal occupies not only the ejection period but also the isovolumic contraction and relaxation periods, is a longer duration signal, and is continuous with the mitral inflow without any intervening gap. The TR signal is similar but tends to be broader with a lower velocity inflow. The cursor position, if visible, is also helpful to identify the origin of the signal. The ventricular septal defect signal is holosystolic but generally tends to have a presystolic component due to LA contraction.

8. **Answer: A.**
   This TEE long axis view of the left atrium and right atrium is also popularly called a bicaval view; the left atrium is immediately anterior to the esophagus.

9. **Answer: A.**
   In a vertical or near vertical plane, the right side is cephalad and the left side is caudal.

10. **Answer: B.**
    Right atrial appendage.

11. **Answer: C.**
    This figure shows pericardial effusion with features of tamponade (right atrial collapse).

12. **Answer: B.**
    Abnormal LV relaxation pattern includes prolonged LV isovolumic relaxation time (> 100 ms), E/A ratio < 1, and E-wave deceleration time > 250 ms.

13. **Answer: A.**
    The arrow denotes the S1 wave, which is caused by LA relaxation. RV ejection and mitral annular descent generate the S2 wave, which follows the S1 wave. The mitral valve opening generates the D-wave, which is synchronous with the mitral E-wave.

14. **Answer: A.**
    The timing of the signal starts with the QRS complex and the end, being continuous with the onset of mitral inflow, suggests MR. A density approaching that of mitral inflow suggests this to be severe. Other clues to severe MR could be a "V-wave cutoff sign" and mitral inflow suggestive of high LA pressure.

15. **Answer: A.**
    The presence of an A-wave excludes atrial fibrillation, mitral stenosis, and prosthetic mitral valve. The E-wave deceleration will be slow. The inflow pattern shown here indicates high LA pressure typified by E/A ratio > 2 and E-wave deceleration of < 150 ms and is consistent with severe MR.

16. **Answer: C.**
    This patient has native aortic valve endocarditis with an anterior aortic ring abscess shown by the arrow. In patients with aortic valve endocarditis it is imperative to look for aortic root, ring, or the mitral–aortic intervalvular fibrosa. TEE is superior to transthoracic echocardiogram for this purpose.

17. **Answer: D.**
    Bicuspid with conjoint left and noncoronary cusps.

18. **Answer: A.**
    Note the membrane attached to the ventricular septum beneath the aortic valve. This is thin and uniformly membranous in appearance.

19. **Answer: A.**
    The systolic signal does not begin with the onset of QRS, which is typical of MR or TR. Hence this is indicative of aortic stenosis (AS) with aortic regurgitation (AR).

The AS signal is midpeaking, which correlates with a slow rise in aortic pressure, as the kinetic energy associated with the jet is very significant and this results in a corresponding drop in potential energy. Note that the end of the AS signal is continuous with the AR signal and vice versa. This indicates the origin of the signals at the same valve.

20. **Answer: C.**

Note the rapid deceleration of the AR signal and that the late diastolic gradient between LV and aorta is only 16 mmHg when applying the simplified Bernoulli equation to the late diastolic AR velocity.

13

Questions

1. This patient is likely to have:

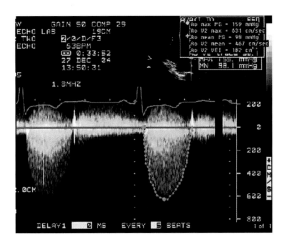

A. Severe aortic stenosis (AS)
B. Severe mitral regurgitation (MR)
C. Severe pulmonary hypertension
D. Mild AS

2. For the patient in Question 1 the left ventricular outflow tract (LVOT) diameter was 2 cm and the LVOT velocity by pulse Doppler was 1 m/s. The aortic valve area by the continuity equation would be:

Echocardiography Board Review: 600 Multiple Choice Questions with Discussion, Third Edition.
Ramdas G. Pai and Padmini Varadarajan.
© 2025 John Wiley & Sons Ltd. Published 2025 by John Wiley & Sons Ltd.

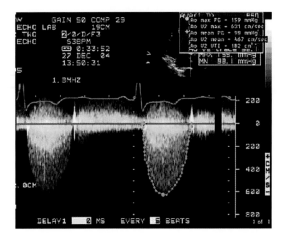

A. 0.2 cm²
B. 0.3 cm²
C. 0.5 cm²
D. 0.8 cm²

3. The image of the aortic arch shown here is indicative of:

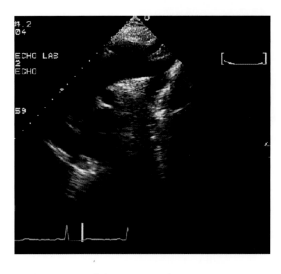

A. Aneurysm of the aortic arch
B. Aortic dissection
C. Severe coarctation of the aorta
D. Stented aortic coarctation

4. This is the continuous wave signal obtained from the pulmonary valve at the mid to proximal esophageal location. This patient is likely to have:

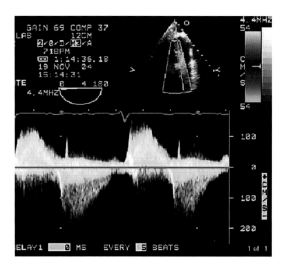

A. Wide open pulmonary regurgitation (PR)
B. Mild PR
C. Severe valvular pulmonary stenosis (PS)
D. Severe subvalvular PS

5. This patient has vegetation on:

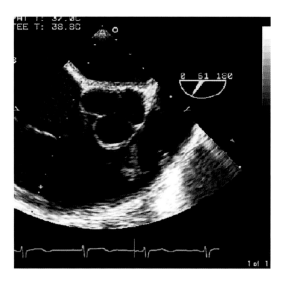

A. Aortic valve
B. Pulmonary valve
C. Tricuspid valve
D. Pacemaker lead

6. The appearance of the left atrial cavity is caused by:

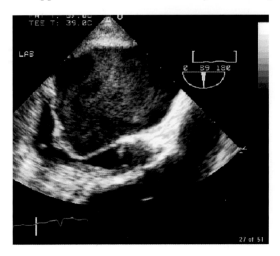

   A. Stasis of blood
   B. MR
   C. Polycythemia
   D. Hyperdynamic circulation

7. The cause of the patient's mitral valve problem is:

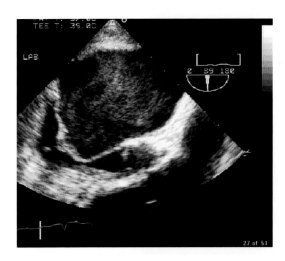

   A. Rheumatic heart disease
   B. Degenerative valve disease
   C. Fen-phen valvulopathy
   D. Ischemic heart disease

8. The arrow in this image points to:

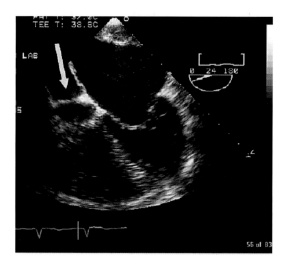

    A. Right atrium (RA)
    B. Coronary sinus
    C. Left atrium (LA)
    D. Right ventricle (RV)

9. The arrow in this image points to:
    A. Left ventricular (LV) apical thrombus
    B. RV thrombus
    C. Rib artifact
    D. LA thrombus

10. This patient is likely to have:

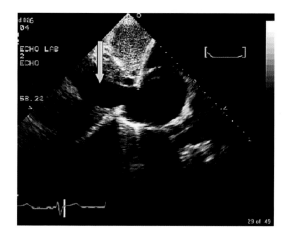

    A. High RA pressure
    B. Pericardial effusion

C. Aortic dissection

D. Dilated azygos vein

11. The pulmonary vein flow shown here is indicative of:

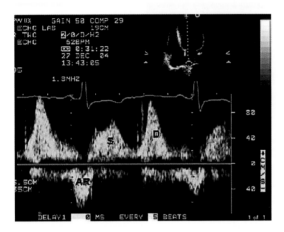

A. Elevated LA pressure with normal end diastolic pressure (EDP)

B. Elevated LA pressure with elevated EDP

C. Abnormal LV relaxation with normal EDP

D. Elevated LVEDP with normal LA pressure

12. The mitral flow pattern shown here is suggestive of:

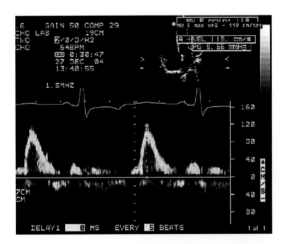

A. Normal LA pressure

B. High LA pressure

C. Atrial mechanical failure

D. Abnormal LV relaxation with normal LA pressure

13. This patient has:

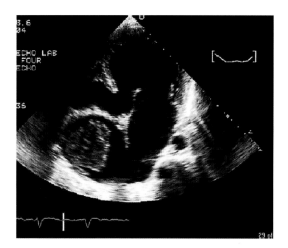

   A. Mitral atresia
   B. Tricuspid atresia
   C. Transposition of great vessels with atrial baffle
   D. Epstein's anomaly

14. The structure denoted by the arrow is likely to be:

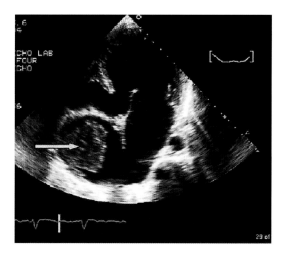

   A. Artifact
   B. Right atrial thrombus
   C. Myxoma
   D. Fibroelastoma

15. This patient is likely to have:

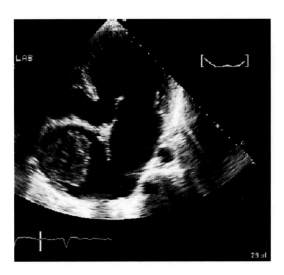

 A. Normal pulmonary artery (PA) flow
 B. Pulmonary hypertension approaching systemic pressure
 C. Nonsignificant amount of flow from RV to PA
 D. None of the above

16. This patient has:

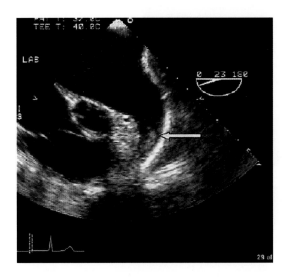

 A. Normal LA appendage
 B. Clot in the LA appendage
 C. Tumor in the LA appendage
 D. None of the above

17. This patient has:

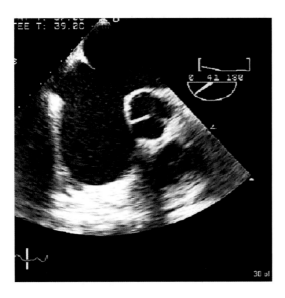

A. Prominent Eustachian valve
B. Ostium secundum atrial septal defect (ASD)
C. Ostium primum ASD
D. Sinus venosus ASD

18. What type of flow was recorded from the mid-esophageal position?

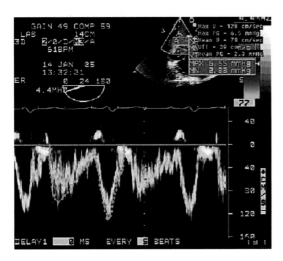

A. Mitral flow
B. Pulmonary vein flow
C. Superior vena cava flow
D. Flow across ASD

19. This patient has a secundum ASD with dimensions of the defect 3 cm × 2 cm, time velocity integral (TVI) of flow across the defect is 39 cm, and the heart rate is 70 beats per minute. The approximate shunt flow across the ASD is:

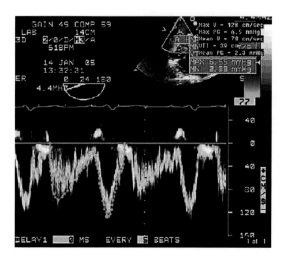

   A. 12.8 L/min
   B. 3 L/min
   C. 7 L/min
   D. Cannot be calculated

20. This patient has:

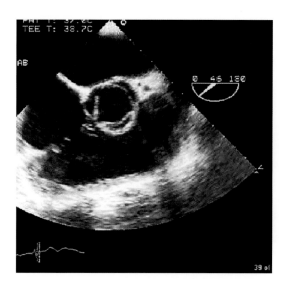

   A. AS
   B. Normal opening trileaflet aortic valve
   C. Bicuspid aortic valve that opens well
   D. Unicommissural aortic valve

Answers for Chapter 13

1. **Answer: A.**
   This is an AS signal. Pay attention to the onset of the signal, which occurs some-
   time after the onset of QRS indicative of signal arising during ejection. Typically a
   peak gradient of > 64 mmHg and a mean gradient of 40 mmHg are indicative of
   severe AS, although these are flow dependent. Valve area is a better indicator of
   severity of AS. MR signal starts with QRS. TR signal in severe pulmonary
   hypertension also starts with QRS.

2. **Answer: C.**
   By the continuity equation $A_1V_1 = A_2V_2$. Hence the aortic valve area $(A_2 = A_1V_1/V_2) =$
   $3.14 \times 1 \times 1 \times 1/6 = 0.5\,cm^2$ approximately.

3. **Answer: D.**
   Note the increased density of the aortic wall in the area of coarctation. This represents the stent.

4. **Answer: A.**
   Note the rapid deceleration of the PR signal with rapid equilibration of late diastolic PA and RV pressures. The increased systolic flow velocity is due to increased
   flow secondary to wide open PR. Note that from this transesophageal echocardiogram (TEE) view you are looking at the pulmonary valve from above, that is, the
   PA side, unlike the parasternal short axis view.

5. **Answer: B.**
   Pulmonary valve. This is an inflow/outflow view of the RV with aortic valve in
   the middle, tricuspid valve on the left of the panel, and pulmonary valve at the
   bottom.

6. **Answer: A.**
   This is a spontaneous echo contrast (smoke like echo, frequently called smoke),
   indicating low velocity of flow, predisposes to thrombus formation, and is a
   marker of embolic risk. Intensity of spontaneous echo contrast is affected by the
   velocity of blood flow and is exaggerated with higher gain settings and a higher
   transducer frequency. Also note the layered thrombus in the body of the LA (at the
   top of the figure).

7. **Answer: A.**
   The patient has classic rheumatic mitral stenosis. The anterior leaflet is thin with
   a hockey-stick appearance in diastole, which occurs due to commissural fusion. In
   degenerative MS there is severe annular calcification, which extends into the leaflets causing stenosis. In fen-phen valvulopathy leaflets are thick and fibrosed and
   may result in both MS and MR. Ischemic involvement of the LV without papillary
   muscle rupture causes restriction of closure and functional MR and not mitral
   stenosis.

8. **Answer: A.**
   RA, to the RA septum.

9. **Answer: A.**
   The position of the septal leaflet of the tricuspid valve confirms the chamber in
   question to be the left ventricle. There is an apical thrombus. The tricuspid valve
   goes with the RV and is more apically placed than the mitral valve.

10. **Answer: A.**
    The inferior vena cava (IVC) as confirmed by its connection to the RA is dilated and is about 2.5 cm in diameter. This indicates high RA pressure; especially if associated with reduced collapse with inspiration. Patients on ventilators may have a dilated IVC without high RA pressure. Young patients might have a dilated IVC with collapse on inspiration, which is normal.

11. **Answer: B.**
    The rapid D-wave deceleration with time < 170 ms indicates high LA pressure. In addition, the S-wave is smaller than the D-wave. The atrial regurgitation (AR) wave duration is about 220 ms. The normal duration is about 80–100 ms. This is due to increased duration of atrial systole having to pump against elevated LVEDP. Pulmonary vein AR duration greater than mitral A-wave duration is indicative of high LVEDP.

12. **Answer: B.**
    This inflow pattern shows a high E/A ratio. The deceleration time is also short, suggestive of high LA pressure. In pure atrial mechanical failure the E-wave is normal, with diminished mitral A-wave amplitude.

13. **Answer: B.**
    The atretic tricuspid valve is shown. There was no ASD, and outflow from RA was through RA to PA shunt. The patient also had a superior vena caval–right PA shunt. Both were patent.

14. **Answer: B.**
    Right atrial thrombus in this patient with tricuspid atresia. Because of atriopulmonary shunt, there is right atrial stasis.

15. **Answer: C.**
    There is tricuspid atresia and pulmonary flow is occurring through cavopulmonary or atriopulmonary shunt in the absence of an ASD. This would need low pulmonary vascular resistance and low PA pressure. This patient has a nonrestrictive ventricular septal defect and hence RV systolic pressure would be the same as LV systolic pressure, and to maintain low PA pressure the RV outflow should be minimal or nonexistent. In this patient this was accomplished surgically with banding of the PA.

16. **Answer: B.**
    This patient has a clot in the LA appendage. This is best visualized with a TEE from an upper esophageal location. The appendage may be multilobed and it is important to examine it in multiple tomographic planes.

17. **Answer: B.**
    Ostium secundum ASD. Primum ASD would be in the lower part of the septum and may involve anterior mitral leaflet and A–V conduction. Sinus venosus ASD is in the upper septum near the superior vena cava and may also be associated with anomalous drainage of the right upper pulmonary vein. There is also a rare type of sinus venosus ASD in the vicinity of the IVC. In unroofed coronary sinus, the shunt is from LA to RA through a posterior defect into the coronary sinus, such that flow goes through the coronary sinus into the RA.

18. **Answer: D.**

    This biphasic flow with a systolic–early diastolic component and LA contraction is typical of ASD flow. Pulmonary vein flow and superior vena cava flow would be triphasic, with distinct systolic and diastolic flows with reversal and atrial contraction. Mitral flow has only diastolic components with early and late diastolic components.

19. **Answer: A.**

    The shunt flow per beat can be calculated as the product of the TVI of the shunt flow and the anatomic area of the defect. This would be $39 \times 3.14 \times 1.5 \times 1$ cc/beat (183 cc). This multiplied by the heart rate gives the shunt flow per minute.

20. **Answer: B.**

    Normal opening of the trileaflet aortic valve.

14

Questions

1. The arrow points to:

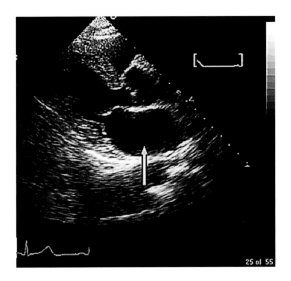

A. Left atrium
B. Right pulmonary artery
C. Posterior pericardial effusion
D. Left pleural effusion

Echocardiography Board Review: 600 Multiple Choice Questions with Discussion, Third Edition.
Ramdas G. Pai and Padmini Varadarajan.
© 2025 John Wiley & Sons Ltd. Published 2025 by John Wiley & Sons Ltd.

2. The structure denoted by the arrow is:

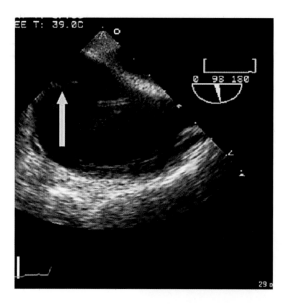

A. Vegetation
B. Eustachian valve
C. Edge of atrial septal defect (ASD)
D. Tricuspid valve

3. The structure shown by the arrow is:

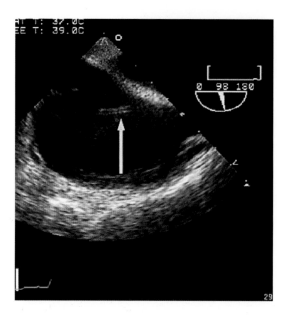

    A. Artifact
    B. Catheter in right atrium
    C. Thrombus
    D. Loose suture material

4. The patient may have all of the following except:

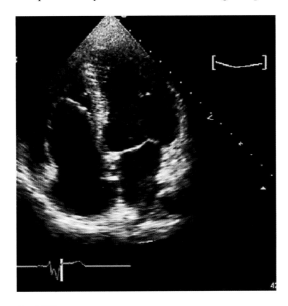

    A. ASD
    B. Wolf–Parkinson–White syndrome
    C. Tricuspid regurgitation
    D. Bicuspid aortic valve

5. The mitral valve abnormality seen here is:

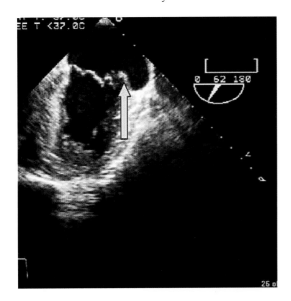

A. Perforation, prolapse of P1 scallop of posterior leaflet
B. Abnormal P3 scallop
C. Prolapsing P2 scallop
D. Anterior leaflet prolapse

6. The structure denoted here is:

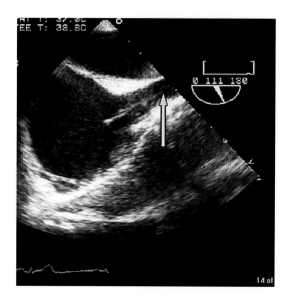

A. Superior vena cava
B. Inferior vena cava (IVC)
C. Right upper pulmonary vein
D. Main pulmonary artery

7. The numbers 1, 2, and 3 denote the following cusps of the aortic valve:

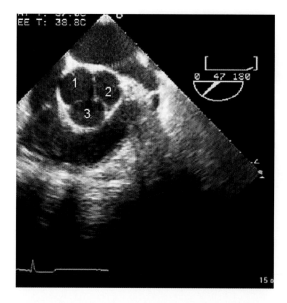

    A. Non-, left, right coronary cusps
    B. Left, right, noncoronary cusps
    C. Right, left, noncoronary cusps
    D. Non-, right, left coronary cusps

8. Structure no. 4 denotes:

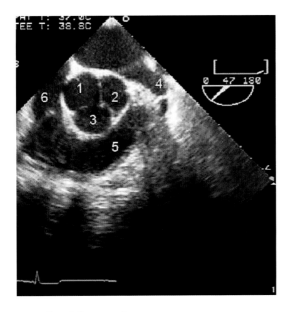

    A. Left atrial appendage
    B. Right atrial appendage
    C. Left upper pulmonary vein
    D. Left lower pulmonary vein

9. The structure shown by the arrow is:

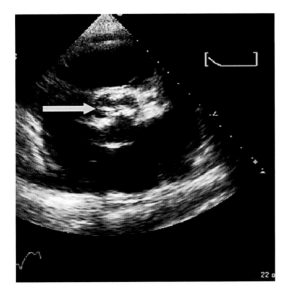

    A. Calcified native aortic valve

    B. Stented bioprosthetic aortic valve

    C. St. Jude bileaflet mechanical aortic valve

    D. Supravalvular aortic stenosis as part of William's syndrome

10. The M-mode echocardiogram is suggestive of:

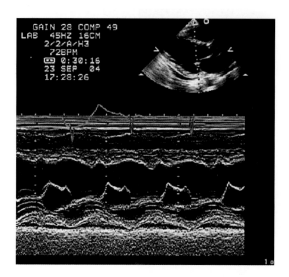

    A. Normal mitral valve motion

    B. Mitral stenosis

    C. Severe aortic regurgitation

    D. High left atrial pressure

11. The image is suggestive of:

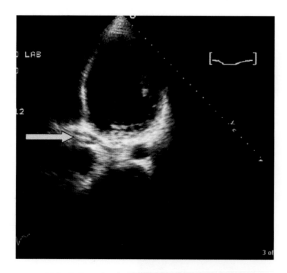

   A. Mitral annuloplasty
   B. Catheter in the coronary artery
   C. Biventricular pacemaker or implantable cardioverter–defibrillator (ICD)
   D. Artifact

12. The structure denoted by the arrow is:

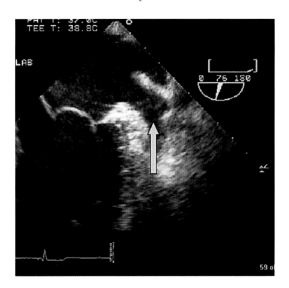

   A. Left atrial appendage
   B. Left lower pulmonary vein
   C. Left upper pulmonary vein
   D. Right lower pulmonary vein

13. The patient shown here has:

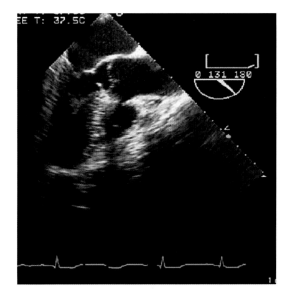

   A. Valvular aortic stenosis
   B. Subvalvular aortic stenosis
   C. Endocarditis
   D. Hypertrophic obstructive cardiomyopathy

14. The arrow is indicative of:

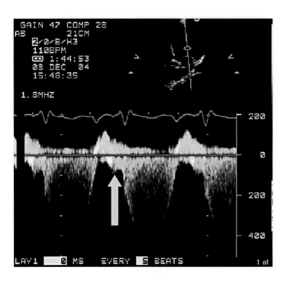

   A. Diastolic mitral regurgitation
   B. Artifact
   C. Pulmonary vein D-wave picked up by the continuous wave cursor
   D. Mitral annular motion superimposed on the mitral flow

15. This patient is likely to have:

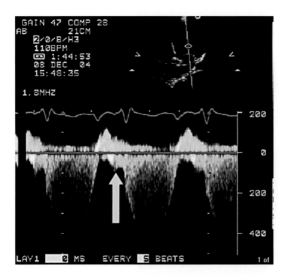

   A. Systolic heart failure
   B. Flail mitral valve with good left ventricular function
   C. Isolated severe acute aortic regurgitation
   D. None of the above

16. This patient is likely to have:

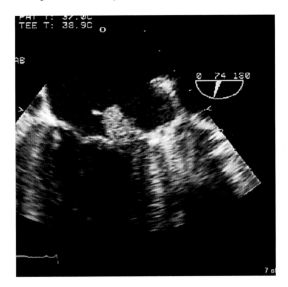

   A. Papillary muscle rupture
   B. Mitral valve endocarditis
   C. Fibroelastoma
   D. Libman–Sacks endocarditis

17. The need for surgical intervention in this patient is:

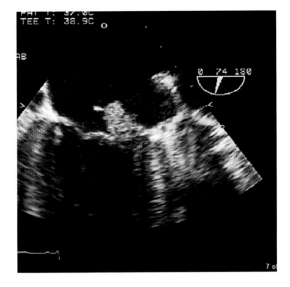

A. Low
B. Intermediate
C. High
D. This is a nonsurgical condition

18. The structure denoted by the arrow is:

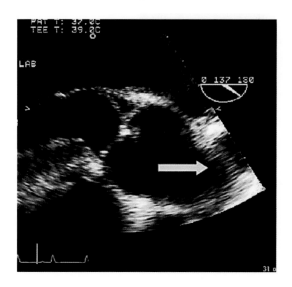

A. Ascending aorta
B. Main pulmonary artery
C. Right atrium
D. Right ventricular outflow tract

19. The structure indicated by the arrow is:

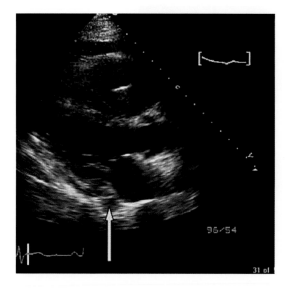

A. Descending thoracic aorta
B. Coronary sinus
C. IVC
D. Circumflex coronary artery

20. The arrow indicates:

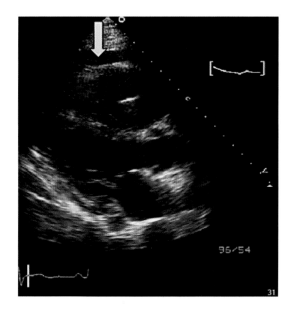

A. Pleural effusion
B. Pericardial effusion
C. Pericardial pad of fat
D. Artifact

Answers for Chapter 14

1. **Answer: A.**
   Left atrium.

2. **Answer: B.**
   The structure is the Eustachian valve. In the vertical plane the IVC is caudal and gets displayed to the left side of the monitor.

3. **Answer: B.**
   This structure has a double wall with a central lumen, which is suggestive of a catheter. In addition the structure is linear. Suture material will not have a lumen and thrombus is not uniform in diameter and has no central lucency.

4. **Answer: D.**
   The patient has Ebstein's anomaly. Note that the downward displacement of the septal leaflet of the tricuspid valve compared to the mitral leaflet attachment. A displacement of > 8 mm/m² is suggestive of Ebstein's anomaly. The septal leaflet may be large, sail like, and adherent to the ventricular septum. This is frequently associated with ASD, right sided accessory pathway, and tricuspid regurgitation, but not bicuspid aortic valve.

5. **Answer: A.**
   In this intercommissural view obtained at about 70 degrees, the area denoted by the arrow is the lateral or P1 scallop of the posterior mitral leaflet. P3 is at the medial commissure. Generally the A2 scallop – that is, the middle scallop of the anterior leaflet – is seen in the middle. However, if the probe is rotated counter-clockwise to the left the P2 scallop may be seen in this location.

6. **Answer: A.**
   This is a long axis image through the superior vena cava (SVC) and the right atrium. Also note a pacing lead in the SVC. Advancing the probe further down the esophagus will show the bicaval view. The left atrium is seen closer to the transducer, separated by the atrial septum from the right atrium. Rightward or clockwise rotation will display the right upper pulmonary vein, and leftward or counterclockwise rotation will show the ascending aorta.

7. **Answer: A.**
   Note that the probe is in the esophagus and the anterior is away from the transducer, contrary to the short axis view of the aortic valve by TEE.

8. **Answer: A.**
   This structure is the left atrial appendage. Structure no. 5 is the right ventricular outflow tract and structure no. 6 is the right atrium.

9. **Answer: A.**
   This is a calcified native aortic valve. The native leaflets are seen. There are no struts of a bioprosthetic valve visible. A mechanical valve produces intense shadowing with poor visualization of the disc unless an end-on view is obtained.

10. **Answer: A.**
    This M mode is suggestive of normal mitral valve motion. There is normal mitral valve opening with greater early diastolic opening compared to opening associated with left atrial contraction. Valvular mitral stenosis would cause

mitral leaflet thickening, reduced opening and reduced ejection fraction (EF) slope, and paradoxical anterior motion of the posterior leaflet during diastole because of commissural fusion. Severe aortic regurgitation (AR) may cause fluttering of the anterior mitral leaflet and premature closure of the anterior mitral leaflet as the mitral valve opening is flow dependent. Features of high left atrial pressure will include predominant early opening, rapid EF slope, and a smaller opening, with atrial contraction mirroring the transmitral inflow pattern.

11. **Answer: C.**
The arrow here depicts a lead in the coronary sinus and is consistent with a biventricular pacemaker.

12. **Answer: A.**
The structure denoted by the arrow is the left atrial appendage. This is separated from the left upper pulmonary vein, which is to the posterior with a ridge popularly known as the "coumadin ridge" because of the potential to be misinterpreted as a thrombus. Because this ridge is echoreflective, sometimes one can see thrombus-like artifacts in the appendage as mirror image artifacts. Though the appendage is clearly visualized here, this view alone is not sufficient to rule out a thrombus. Multiple tomographic views have to be obtained through the appendage in its entirety as the appendage may have multiple lobes.

13. **Answer: B.**
The structure attached to the septum below the aortic valve is a classic subaortic membrane. Occasionally vegetations can be seen here due to seeding from the aortic valve. This is a diastolic frame and hence aortic valve opening cannot be evaluated.

14. **Answer: A.**
This is diastolic mitral regurgitation (MR), which in this patient is probably due to high left ventricular end diastolic pressure (LVEDP) or coexistent severe AR. Other causes of diastolic MR include prolonged PR interval, prolonged A–V delay, or A–V dissociation. The velocity of this signal is about 1.2 m/s, which is high for tissue velocity. The pulmonary vein D-wave would be in the opposite direction, that is, in the direction of the mitral E-wave.

15. **Answer: A.**
The profile of MR is indicative of severe LV systolic dysfunction in view of the prolonged duration of the MR signal and severely reduced dp/dt in the presence of normal QRS duration. In this example the time taken for the MR velocity to rise from 1 to 3 m/s is 60 ms, which translates into an LV positive dp/dt of 530 mmHg/s (32/0.06). Also note that the diastolic filling period is short and the diastolic MR in this patient is likely from high LVEDP, as the PR interval is not unduly prolonged.

16. **Answer: B.**
There is a large mass attached to the P1 scallop of the mitral valve with a soft tissue characteristically less echo dense than the mitral leaflets and a secondary thin mass attached to this. The attachment of this lesion is to the atrial side of the mitral leaflet. This is highly consistent with vegetation. Nonbacterial vegetation of Libman–Sacks endocarditis is a complication of systemic lupus erythematosus and is generally smaller, multiple, and verrucous. Fibroelastomas are more echo dense, nodular, generally pedunculated, and mobile, usually attached to the ventricular side of the mitral valve.

17. **Answer: C.**
    The vegetation is very large, measuring about 1.5×1 cm, and has a high embolic potential in view of its mobility, large size, and mobile elements attached to its tip. It also has a high potential for lack of bacterial clearance with antibiotics alone because of the size. In addition, this patient has severe MR. In general, the indications for surgery include lack of response to medical therapy, valvular disruption, recurrent embolization, abscess formation, and fungal vegetations. Size greater than 1 cm is a relative indication for surgery because of the potential for complications.

18. **Answer: A.**
    Ascending aorta. Also note long vegetation on the aortic valve on its left ventricular side.

19. **Answer: B.**
    This structure is in the posterior A–V groove, is intrapericardial, and is markedly dilated. Dilatation can occur as a result of either increased flow or increased pressure. Causes include persistent left SVC, right heart failure, coronary fistula, and unroofed coronary sinus. Descending thoracic aorta is extrapericardial. Hence, if there is a pericardial effusion, it would be anterior to the aorta and pleural effusion would be posterior to the aorta. This degree of aneurysm of circumflex artery is unusual. The IVC does not course this area.

20. **Answer: B.**
    This echolucent space is clearly between two layers of the pericardium. The space is totally echolucent, which indicates fluid rather than fat tissue. Speckled appearance in this area would be indicative of epicardial pad of fat. Pericardial pad of fat would be outside the parietal pericardium.

15

Questions

1. This image shows a vegetation on the:

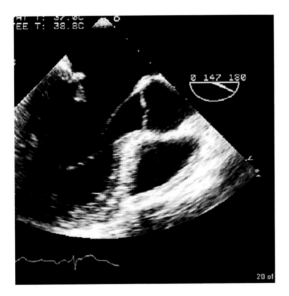

A. Aortic valve
B. P2 scallop of mitral valve
C. P1 scallop of mitral valve
D. A2 scallop of mitral valve

Echocardiography Board Review: 600 Multiple Choice Questions with Discussion, Third Edition.
Ramdas G. Pai and Padmini Varadarajan.
© 2025 John Wiley & Sons Ltd. Published 2025 by John Wiley & Sons Ltd.

2. The hemodynamics in this patient potentially could be improved by:

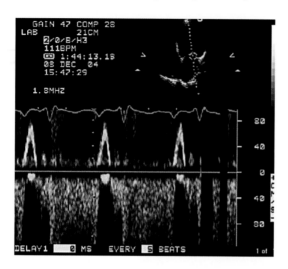

   A. Shortening the PR interval
   B. Afterload reduction
   C. Positive inotropes
   D. All of the above

3. The transesophageal echocardiogram (TEE) image shown here is indicative of:

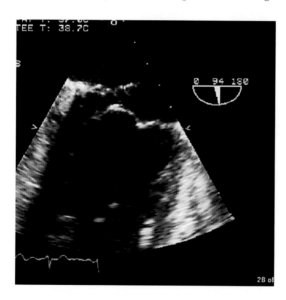

   A. Flail posterior leaflet P3 segment
   B. Flail posterior leaflet P1 segment

C. Flail anterior leaflet

D. Large mitral valve vegetation

4. The pulse wave Doppler in the right upper pulmonary vein is indicative of:

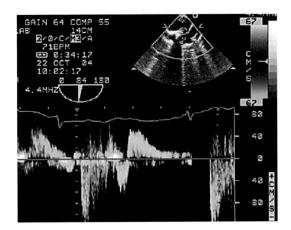

A. Abnormal left ventricular (LV) relaxation

B. High left atrial (LA) pressure

C. Mitral stenosis

D. Severe mitral regurgitation (MR)

5. This apical four-chamber view shows:

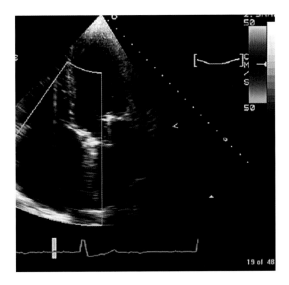

A. A pacemaker lead in the right ventricle (RV)

B. A pacemaker lead in the coronary sinus

    C. Epicardial RV lead

    D. Artifact in the RV

6. The mitral valve opening pattern in this patient is suggestive of:

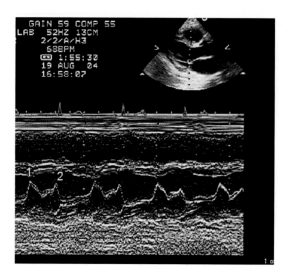

    A. Mitral stenosis

    B. High left ventricular end diastolic pressure (LVEDP)

    C. Atrial fibrillation

    D. Normal pattern

7. The part of the anatomy and measurement indicated by the line is:

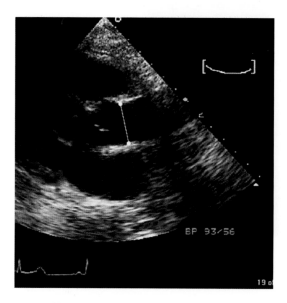

    A. The sino-tubular junction
    B. Sinus diameter
    C. Sinus height
    D. Aortic annular diameter

8. The blood supply to the ventricular septum shown here is:

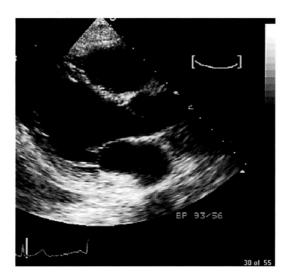

    A. Left anterior descending (LAD) artery
    B. Posterior descending artery
    C. Both of the above
    D. Neither of the above

9. The structure indicated by the arrow in the ascending aorta is likely to be:

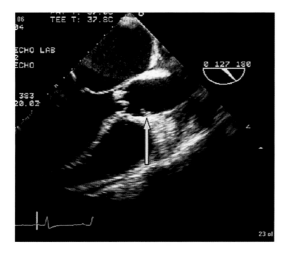

    A. Vegetative aortitis
    B. Flap of aortic dissection
    C. Intraaortic atherosclerotic debris
    D. Supravalvular aortic stenosis

10. The structure indicated by the arrow is likely to be:

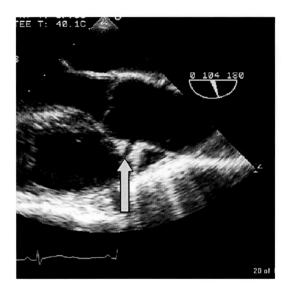

    A. Aortic dissection
    B. Aortic transaction
    C. Right coronary artery
    D. Left coronary artery

11. The arrow in this short axis view transthoracic echocardiogram (TTE) image at the level of the ascending aorta is:

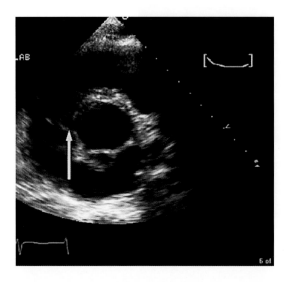

A. Artifact
B. Tissue plane and aorta and RV outflow tract
C. Aortic dissection
D. Right coronary artery

12. The structure shown by the arrow is:

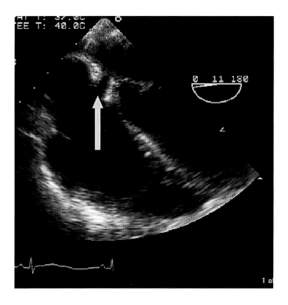

A. Coronary sinus
B. Atrial septal defect (ASD)
C. Superior vena cava
D. Inferior vena cava

13. The valve indicated by the arrow is:

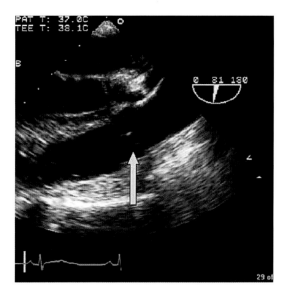

A. Pulmonary valve
B. Aortic valve
C. Tricuspid valve
D. Mirror image artifact of the aortic valve

14. This view is obtained from the upper esophagus. The structure indicated by the arrow is:

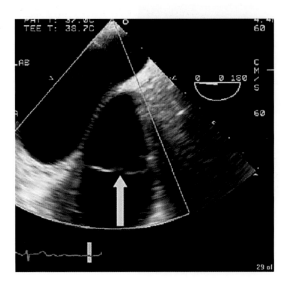

A. Aortic valve
B. Pulmonary valve
C. Tricuspid valve
D. Artifact

15. The pulmonary regurgitation signal shown here is indicative of (assuming right atrial pressure of 15 mmHg):

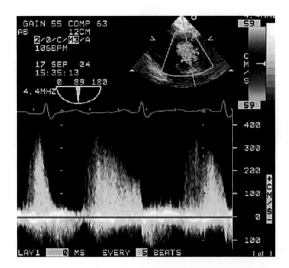

    A. Normal pulmonary artery (PA) pressure

    B. Mild pulmonary hypertension

    C. Moderate pulmonary hypertension

    D. None of the above

16. This subcostal view shows part of the liver. This patient has a history of episodes of flushing and diarrhea. The likely diagnosis is:

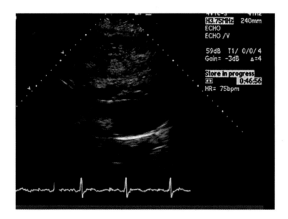

    A. Amebic liver abscess

    B. Right atrial myxoma

    C. Carcinoid syndrome

    D. Renal cell carcinoma

17. This 86-year-old patient has intractable heart failure and chronic atrial fibrillation. The finding on the still image is suggestive of:

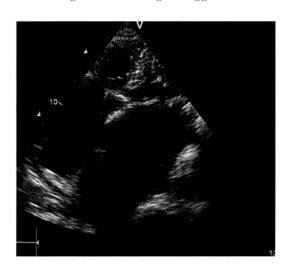

    A. LA thrombus

    B. Lipomatous atrial septum

    C. ASD closure device

    D. Side lobe artifact

18. In Question 17 the LV size and ejection fraction were normal. The patient is likely to have:

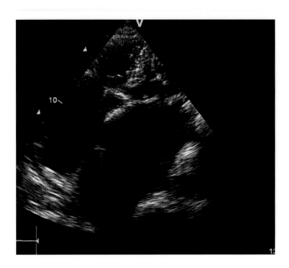

    A. Restrictive cardiomyopathy

    B. Congestive cardiomyopathy

    C. Hypertrophic cardiomyopathy

    D. None of the above

19. The short axis image of this patient shows:

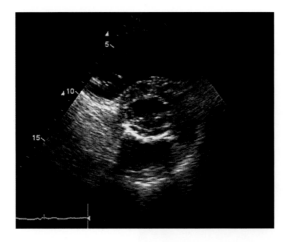

    A. Posterior pericardial effusion

    B. Massive mitral annular calcification

    C. Calcified aortic valves

    D. None of the above

20. The appearance of the interatrial septum is indicative of:

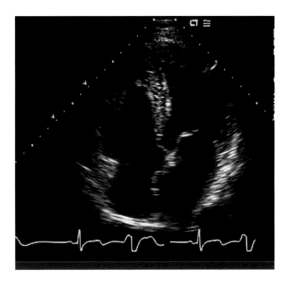

A. LA myxoma
B. Aneurysmal atrial septum
C. ASD
D. None of the above

Answers for Chapter 15

1. **Answer: B.**
   This is a long axis cut through the mitral valve, which courses through the middle of both the anterior and posterior leaflets and hence would show A2 and P2 scallops, respectively. Pushing the probe down will cut through A3 and P3 scallops and pulling the probe up will cut through A1 and P1 scallops.

2. **Answer: D.**
   Note that this patient has a markedly dilated LV and very short diastole despite a heart rate of about 70/min, very premature atrial contraction with no passive transmitral flow, with diastolic MR and prolonged systole as indicated by the systolic MR signal. All of these indicate poor systolic performance and AV dyssynchrony. Hence the hemodynamics is likely to improve with the therapies listed. The QRS duration in the monitored ECG is 100 ms. However, the 12-lead ECG has to be examined for QRS duration. If QRS duration is prolonged, or mechanical asynchrony is demonstrated by echocardiography, then the patient may also benefit from biventricular pacing.

3. **Answer: A.**
   This patient has a flail P3 scallop of the posterior mitral leaflet. In this near intercommissural view, with slight rightward rotation, the scallops from right to left include A1, A2, and P3. At about a 70–80 degree angle the scallops seen would be P1, A2, and P3. At around 120–130 degrees the scallops seen would be A2 and P2.

4. **Answer: D.**
   This is severe MR. Note the holosystolic flow reversal in the pulmonary vein.

5. **Answer: A.**
   This is an RV endocardial lead. The coronary sinus (CS) is not visualized here. The CS lead tends to be thinner. CS can be imaged with a posterior tilt from this plane. The implantable cardioverter–defibrillator (ICD) leads are much thicker than the pacer leads.

6. **Answer: D.**
   This is an M mode through the mitral valve showing a normal pattern with E(1) and A(2) waves on the image of normal amplitude and movement of the posterior leaflet, which is a mirror image in the opposite direction. In atrial fibrillation the A-wave disappears. High LVEDP is classically characterized by a "B" hump, which is a positive deflection on the downslope of the A-wave. Features of mitral stenosis include mitral leaflet thickening, reduced opening, flatter EF slope, and paradoxical anterior motion of the posterior leaflet during diastole due to leaflet fusion.

7. **Answer: A.**
   This is the sino-tubular junction (STJ), which is the junction between the sinus and the tubular portions of the ascending aorta. This diameter is usually less than the annulus diameter. The sinus height is the distance between the annulus and the STJ and is increased in conditions that cause aneurysmal dilatation of the sinus portion of the aorta. Excessive dilatation of the STJ may cause restriction in the closure of the aortic valve and may result in aortic regurgitation in the absence of leaflet pathology and in the presence of normal annulus size. This can be corrected by restoration of the aortic root anatomy with root replacement.

8. **Answer: A.**
   The entire ventricular septum seen here is anterior, supplied by the LAD artery. The first septal perforator of the LAD artery supplies the very proximal septum.

9. **Answer: A.**
   This thin filamentous mass in association with aortic valve vegetation was vegetation on the aortic wall seeding the right side of the aortic wall as a jet lesion. There is no false lumen or intramural hematoma to support the diagnosis of a flap. The remainder of the aorta is normal without any atherosclerotic changes; however, a small atheromatous mass is still a possibility.

10. **Answer: C.**
    This is anterior and the artery is coming out of the right sinus of Valsalva on this TEE. Dissection will be characterized by a thin mobile flap and a false lumen. In transection there would be a thicker, localized flap protruding into the aortic lumen associated with disruption of media and adventitia.

11. **Answer: D.**
    Note the tubular nature of the structure and its continuity with the aortic lumen. The right coronary artery (RCA) arises anteriorly from this location and the origin of the left coronary artery would be in the 4 o'clock position (not shown here). Here, the RCA is originating anomalously from the junction of right and noncoronary sinuses.

12. **Answer: A.**
    This low esophageal view at the gastroesophageal junction with the transverse plane in the A–V groove posteriorly demonstrates the coronary sinus draining into the right atrium. A long axis cut through the vena cavae is generally seen in the vertical bicaval view in the 80–120 degree angle.

13. **Answer: A.**
    Note that this is anterior and connects to the PA. Also seen is part of the aortic valve posterior to this structure.

14. **Answer: B.**
    The structure indicated by the arrow is the pulmonary valve. The structure closer to the transducer is the aortic arch in transverse plane. Part of the main PA is seen closer to the transducer. This is a good TEE view for Doppler interrogation of pulmonary valve or main pulmonary artery.

15. **Answer: C.**
    The end diastolic velocity is 2.1 m/s, which translates into an end diastolic gradient of 17 mmHg between the PA and the RV. Assuming the RVEDP to be the same as the mean RA pressure of 15 mmHg, the computed PA end diastolic pressure would be 32 mmHg. This is consistent with moderate to severe pulmonary hypertension. Also note that the PR signal is rapidly decelerating, indicating either severe pulmonary regurgitation or rapidly increasing RVEDP.

16. **Answer: C.**
    The image shows abnormal liver with a multiple echogenic and echoluscent area consistent with metastatic tumor. This combined with the clinical presentation is indicative of carcinoid syndrome. Valves most commonly affected include the tricuspid and pulmonary valves. Renal cell carcinoma may extend to the heart through the inferior vena cava. Right atrial myxoma usually is attached to the atrial septum or the atrial free wall.

17. **Answer: A.**
    This is a left atrial thrombus. A large mass is visualized attached to the atrial septum in the fossa ovalis area. In the given clinical context this is likely to be a thrombus. Differential diagnosis includes left atrial myxoma. Lipomatous atrial septum spares the fossa ovalis but causes thickening of the rest of the septum due to fat deposition. An ASD closure device like the Amplatzer device has a characteristic internal architecture made up of mesh and wires. Note the severely dilated left atrium. This patient was in chronic atrial fibrillation predisposing him to left atrial thrombus formation.

18. **Answer: A.**
    Severe biatrial enlargement with a normal sized ventricle associated with high filling pressures is diagnostic of restrictive cardiomyopathy. This patient has aneurysmal biatrial enlargement. This patient also had low-voltage electrocardiographic complexes, which is suggestive of cardiac amyloidosis.

19. **Answer: B.**
    The posterior annulus is massively calcified. The echolucent area posterior to this is due to shadowing because of lack of penetration through this massively calcified structure.

20. **Answer: B.**
    The fossa ovalis is bowing toward the right atrium. This back-and-forth movement of the fossa is better visualized during dynamic imaging. This is associated with patent foramen ovale and increased risk of stroke and possibly migraine. The image does not show any mass or atrial septal defect, though a tangential cut through the aneurysmal septum may mimic a mass in certain views during dynamic imaging.

16

Questions

1. The parasternal long axis image of the mitral valve apparatus shows:

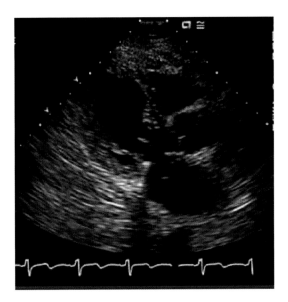

    A. Mitral annular calcification
    B. Rheumatic mitral stenosis
    C. Systolic anterior motion
    D. Annuloplasty ring

Echocardiography Board Review: 600 Multiple Choice Questions with Discussion, Third Edition.
Ramdas G. Pai and Padmini Varadarajan.
© 2025 John Wiley & Sons Ltd. Published 2025 by John Wiley & Sons Ltd.

2. The continuous wave signal with a peak velocity of 3.2 m/s shown here is indicative of:

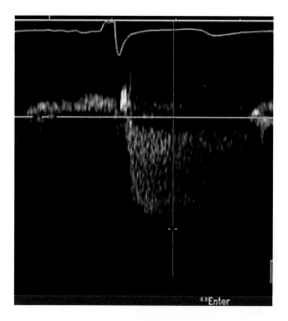

   A. Moderate aortic stenosis
   B. Moderate pulmonary hypertension
   C. Acute severe mitral regurgitation due to papillary muscle rupture
   D. None of the above

3. Assuming a right atrial (RA) pressure of 10 mmHg, the pulmonary regurgitation signal with an end diastolic velocity of 2.2 m/s shown here is indicative of:

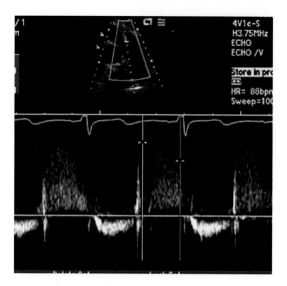

    A. Normal pulmonary artery (PA) pressure

    B. Moderate elevation of PA pressure

    C. Systemic level of PA pressure

    D. None of the above

4. The abnormalities shown in this image include:

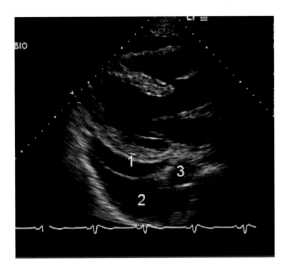

    A. Pericardial effusion

    B. Left pleural effusion

    C. Left pleural effusion and pericardial effusion

    D. Abnormally thick pericardium

5. The pattern of aortic valve opening in this patient is likely to be due to:

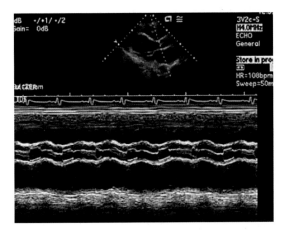

    A. Hypertrophic obstructive cardiomyopathy (HOCM)

    B. Pulsus alternans

C. Intraaortic balloon pump (IABP) with 1:3 support

D. Left ventricular assist device (LVAD) with 1:3 support

6. This is an apical four-chamber view of the left ventricle (LV). The structure indicated by the arrow in the LV apex is likely to be:

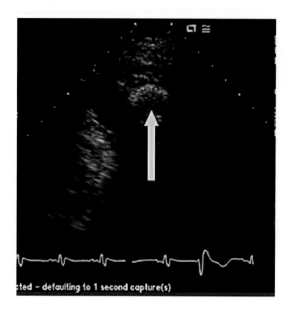

A. LV thrombus

B. Rib artifact

C. Cannula of LVAD

D. False tendon in the LV apex

7. The structure indicated by the arrow is:

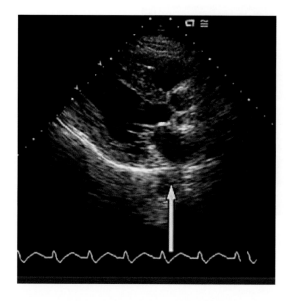

    A. Descending thoracic aorta
    B. Coronary sinus
    C. Left lower pulmonary vein
    D. Left PA

8. The transthoracic image shown here is indicative of:

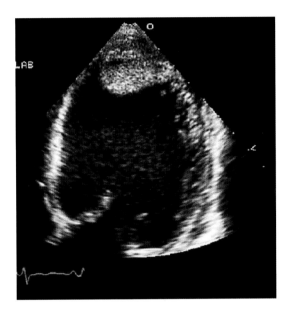

    A. LV apical thrombus
    B. Moderator band
    C. Rib artifact
    D. Ventricular noncompaction

9. The patient shown here is likely to have:

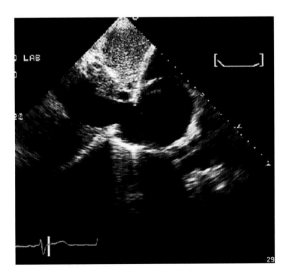

    A. Heart failure

    B. Intravascular volume depletion with hypotension

    C. RA tumor

    D. None of the above

10. The continuous wave Doppler signal shown here is suggestive of:

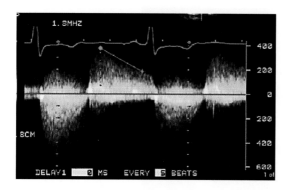

    A. Mixed mitral valve disease with significant mitral stenosis (MS) and mitral regurgitation (MR)

    B. Mixed aortic valve disease with significant aortic stenosis (AS) and aortic regurgitation (AR)

    C. Combination of AR and MR

    D. Ventricular septal defect (VSD) with bidirectional flow

11. This patient (BP 130/65 mmHg) is likely to have:

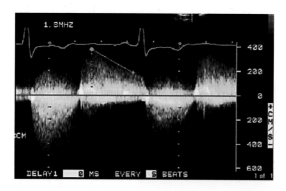

    A. High left ventricular end diastolic pressure (LVEDP)

    B. Diastolic MR

    C. Premature mitral valve closure

    D. All of the above

12. The following statements are true of the Doppler signal shown here:

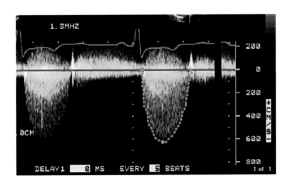

A. The patient may have severe valvular AS
B. The patient may have severe systolic anterior motion (SAM)
C. The patient may have severe MR
D. None of the above

13. The pulmonary vein flow pattern is indicative of:

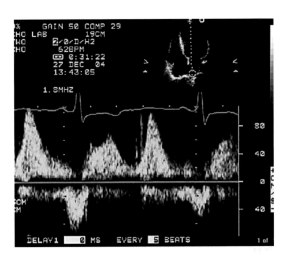

A. Volume depletion
B. Atrial fibrillation
C. Elevated LVEDP with normal left atrial (LA) pressure
D. Elevated LVEDP with high LA pressure

14. This patient has:

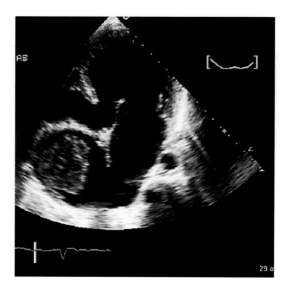

  A. Tricuspid atresia
  B. Right atrial myxoma
  C. Hydatid cyst of the heart
  D. Hypoplastic left heart syndrome

15. The flow shown here is consistent with:

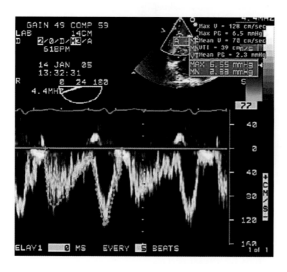

  A. Superior vena cava (SVC) flow
  B. Pulmonary vein flow
  C. Atrial septal defect (ASD) flow
  D. None of the above

16. This patient had secundum ASD fairly circular with a diameter of 2 cm. The heart rate was 61/min. The approximate shunt flow would be:

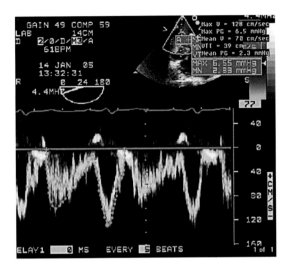

A. 5 L/min
B. 7.4 L/min
C. 13 L/min
D. 20 L/min

17. The abnormality shown in this image could be associated with:

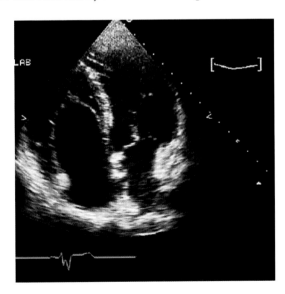

A. Accessory pathway
B. ASD
C. Tricuspid regurgitation
D. All of the above

18. The patient shown here has:

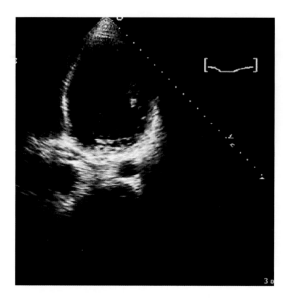

    A. Prosthetic mitral valve
    B. Tricuspid atresia
    C. Left SVC
    D. Biventricular pacemaker

19. The cause of the abnormality shown here could be:

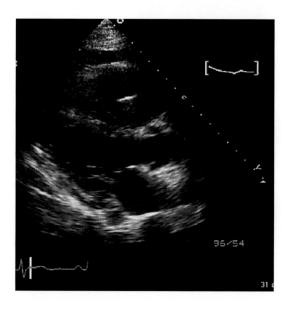

A. Persistent left SVC
B. Congestive heart failure
C. Unroofed coronary sinus
D. All of the above

20. The patient shown here has:

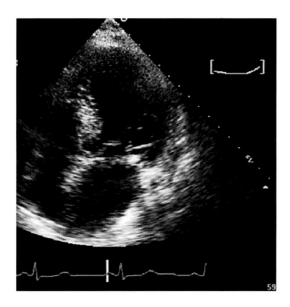

A. Severe mitral annular calcification
B. Mitral annuloplasty ring
C. Rheumatic mitral valve disease
D. None of the above

Answers for Chapter 16

1. **Answer: D.**
   Posterior mitral annuloplasty ring in cross-section. This is circular in cross-section and on the atrial side of the base of the posterior mitral leaflet. Mitral annular calcification on the contrary will bury the leaflet base inside the calcification and generally starts from the base of the annulus and extends to the leaflets, and the shape is not circular in cross-section. There is no restriction of the leaflet tips to suggest rheumatic involvement and SAM is evaluated in systole. This is a diastolic frame.

2. **Answer: B.**
   This is a signal originating from A–V valve regurgitation as it starts with the QRS without any isovolumic contraction. Accompanying forward flow velocity is less than 1/2 m/s, suggesting tricuspid origin. Mitral inflow velocity tends to be higher. The velocity of this signal is 3.2 m/s, resulting in a transvalvular gradient of about 40 mmHg. Assuming an RA pressure of 10 mmHg, the right ventricular (RV) systolic pressure would be 50 mmHg. Aortic signal is of shorter duration and starts later after the isovolumic contraction period and if mitral inflow is visible the isovolumic relaxation time could be discerned, that is, the aortic velocity curve will not be continuous with the mitral inflow velocity curve. In acute severe MR, the gradient could be low due to hypotension and high LA pressure. In such a situation, a large V-wave would result in rapid deceleration of the signal soon after finishing acceleration. This is the so-called V-wave "cutoff" sign.

3. **Answer: B.**
   End diastolic pulmonary regurgitation velocity is 2 m/s, consistent with a PA to RV end diastolic gradient of 16 mmHg (4×2^2). Assuming that the RV end diastolic pressure is close to the mean RA pressure, the PA diastolic pressure will be 26 mmHg.

4. **Answer: C.**
   Number 1 indicates pericardial effusion, 2 indicates pleural effusion, and 3 is the descending aorta. Pericardial effusion is always anterior to the aorta and pleural effusion extends posteriorly. The structure separating the two is combined parietal pericardium and pleura. The combined thickness is < 3 mm, which is normal.

5. **Answer: D.**
   There is reduced aortic valve opening with every third beat. This is due to reduced transaortic flow with every third beat, which is assisted by the LVAD, and the bulk of the cardiac output is delivered through the assist device. During the intervening two beats, all the stroke volume is delivered through the aortic valve. With 1:3 IABP support the increase in stroke volume during the IABP deflation occurs through the aortic valve, hence there is increased opening. In pulsus alternans, strong and weak beats alternate in a 1:2 fashion. In HOCM, midsystolic closure occurs with every beat.

6. **Answer: C.**
   Echodense walls and echoluscent lumen of the cannula are seen. This LVAD cannula serves to deliver blood to the assist device. In these patients it is important to make sure that there is no obstruction to the inlet cannula by surrounding structures, including the ventricular septum, and no apical thrombi. Thrombus does not have a central lucency. False tendons are echodense and linear and rib artifacts are lighter and generally go through the anatomic boundaries.

7. **Answer: A.**

   This vessel is posterior to the left atrium, indicative of descending thoracic aorta. Coronary sinus is in the posterior A–V groove and is intrapericardial. The left PA and the left lower pulmonary vein are far away from this location.

8. **Answer: A.**

   An LV apical thrombus. There is a distinctly demarcated thrombus in the apex. When there is a question, this can be confirmed by obtaining additional views of the apex, such as two-chamber and short axis views with color flow imaging at a low Nyquist limit or using transpulmonary contrast agents such as Definity, when a thrombus will be seen as a filling defect. The LV apex is a common place for a false tendon and may be mistaken for a thrombus. Rib artifact is less dense, goes beyond the endocardium, and does not move with the heart.

9. **Answer: A.**

   Heart failure. Dilated inferior vena cava (IVC) is suggestive of high RA pressure if it does not collapse with inspiration. Occasionally in normal young individuals one may see a dilated IVC, which readily collapses with inspiration. A general guideline is that IVC > 2 cm and < 10% collapse indicates RA pressure > 20 mmHg; > 2 cm and 50% collapse indicates RA pressure of 15 mmHg; 1.5–2 cm and > 50% collapse indicates RA pressure of 10 mmHg; and < 1 cm and > 50% collapse indicates RA pressure of 5 mmHg. However, new American Society of Echocardiography (ASE) guidelines are as follows: IVC $\leq$ 2.1 cm and > 50% collapse with a sniff is suggestive of normal RA pressure of 3 mmHg (range 0–5 mmHg). IVC $\geq$ 2.1 cm and < 50% collapse is suggestive of high RA pressure, 15 mmHg (range 10–20 mmHg). In indeterminate cases the size of the IVC and collapse do not fit this paradigm, so an intermediate value of 8 mmHg (range 5–10 mmHg) may be used. Alternately, secondary indices of high RA pressure should be integrated such as tricuspid E/E′ > 6, diastolic flow predominance in the hepatic veins. In indeterminate cases, if secondary indices of elevated RA pressure are not present, RA pressure can be downgraded to 3 mmHg. If there is minimal IVC collapse with a sniff (< 35%) and secondary indices of high RA pressure are present, then RA pressure can be upgraded to 15 mmHg. If uncertain, leave RA pressure at 8 mmHg. In patients who are unable to perform a sniff, an IVC that collapses < 20% with quiet respiration suggests high RA pressure. IVC collapse does not accurately reflect RA pressure in ventilator-dependent patients. (J Am Soc Echocardiogr 2010;23:685–713.)

10. **Answer: B.**

    Mixed aortic valve disease with significant AS and AR. Diastolic signal is diagnostic of AR with a 4 m/s early diastolic velocity, which does not occur with MS. The velocity curve of AR is continuous with the systolic signal, indicating signal origin at the same valve. The MR signal would be longer and overlap both the initial and terminal portions of the AR signal, as MR would occur with both isovolumic contraction and relaxation phases. The typical VSD signal will have a systolic component and a presystolic associated with LA contraction directed into the RV. If the patient has Eisenmenger's syndrome, the flow velocity would be very low.

11. **Answer: D.**

    All of the above. The AR signal decelerates rapidly with a pressure half-time of 185 ms (< 250 ms indicates very rapid deceleration). The end diastolic velocity is about 2 ms, indicating an end diastolic gradient between the aorta and LV of

16 mmHg, assuming alignment of the ultrasound beam parallel to flow. As the patient's diastolic pressure is 65 mmHg, the LVEDP is 49 mmHg (65 – 16). Severe AR, generally acute, or significant AR in the presence of stiff LV may occur with severe AS or hypertension; high LVEDP resulting from this may cause diastolic MR and also presystolic closure of the mitral valve.

12. **Answer: A.**
Severe valvular AS. The timing of the onset slightly after the onset of the QRS complex, suggestive of onset after the LV isovolumic contraction period, is suggestive of aortic origin. Although the aortic valve area is the best indicator of AS severity, a mean gradient of > 50 mmHg is generally consistent with severe AS. In addition, the signal is mid to late peaking, which has the same significance as the mid to late peaking of the AS murmur. SAM would cause a dagger-shaped, late-peaking signal because of the dynamic nature of the obstruction.

13. **Answer: D.**
Elevated LVEDP with high LA pressure. The D-wave velocity, which is higher than the S-wave velocity with rapid deceleration (time < 170 ms), is indicative of high LA pressure in an adult. Small S and large D could be normal in children because of very efficient LV relaxation. In the example shown here, the AR-wave duration is markedly increased. Normally, AR-wave duration is less than mitral A-wave duration and is < 110–120 ms. Although A-wave duration is not shown here, the AR-wave duration is grossly abnormal at 200 ms, indicating high LVEDP, causing an increase in the duration of atrial systole because of increased atrial afterload. In a volume-depleted patient the S-wave will be prominent and the AR-wave would be diminutive; in atrial fibrillation, the AR-wave is lost.

14. **Answer: A.**
Tricuspid atresia. The image shows an absent tricuspid valve, a right atrial mass that is consistent and likely to be a thrombus due to stasis, and a VSD. This patient had cavopulmonary anastomosis with SVC–RPA (right pulmonary artery) and RA–LPA (left pulmonary artery) shunt such that IVC blood drained into the LPA through the RA, causing thrombus formation. The PA was completely banded to facilitate cavopulmonary flow. This patient has a well-developed left heart and hence does not have hypoplastic left heart syndrome. Right atrial myxoma is a possibility, but thrombus is much more likely in this situation.

15. **Answer: C.**
ASD flow. The flow shown is typical of ASD flow with systolic–diastolic wave and a second wave associated with atrial contraction, all left to right in the same direction. Both SVC and pulmonary vein flows are triphasic with S-, D-, and AR-waves, with the AR-wave being in an opposite direction to the S- and D-waves.

16. **Answer: B.**
7.4 L/min. The shunt flow per heart beat is the time velocity integral (TVI) across the defect × cross-sectional area, that is, $39 \times 3.14 \times 1 \times 1 = 122$ cc (TVI of signal is 39 cm). Shunt flow per minute = shunt volume per beat × heart rate = $122 \times 61 = 7.4$ L/min.

17. **Answer: D.**
The image is diagnostic of Ebstein's anomaly of the tricuspid valve. This is diagnosed when the attachment of the septal leaflet of the tricuspid valve is apically displaced in relation to the anterior leaflet by > 8 mm/m². In this disorder the

septal leaflet is large, sail like, and could be plastered to the RV wall through the chordae tendinae. The associations include severe tricuspid regurgitation, ASD, and right-sided accessory pathway causing paroxysmal supraventricular tachycardia.

18. **Answer: D.**

    Biventricular pacemaker. A coronary sinus lead is clearly seen in this image. This is imaged from the apical four-chamber view with a posterior transducer tilt to obtain a tomographic plane through the coronary sinus. Because of this the mitral valve is not seen. The coronary sinus is not enlarged to support the diagnosis of left SVC.

19. **Answer: D.**

    All of the above. The coronary sinus is dilated, which could be due to increased flow or pressure, and any of the conditions listed can potentially result in a dilated coronary sinus. Note that the coronary sinus is in the A–V groove and the intra-pericardial versus descending aorta, which is in the posterior mediastinum and is extrapericardial.

20. **Answer: B.**

    Mitral annuloplasty ring. Echocardiographically, this is distinguished from mitral annular calcification by its rounded shape in cross-section and projection into the left atrium at the base of the posterior leaflet. In contrast, mitral annular calcification would incorporate the base of the posterior mitral leaflet into itself.

17

Questions

1. The cause of dyspnea in this patient is likely to be:

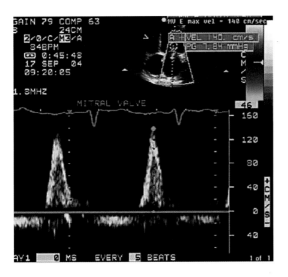

A. Left heart failure
B. Primary pulmonary hypertension
C. Chronic obstructive pulmonary disorder
D. None of the above

2. This is an end systolic frame in a patient with shortness of breath. The most likely diagnosis is:

Echocardiography Board Review: 600 Multiple Choice Questions with Discussion, Third Edition.
Ramdas G. Pai and Padmini Varadarajan.
© 2025 John Wiley & Sons Ltd. Published 2025 by John Wiley & Sons Ltd.

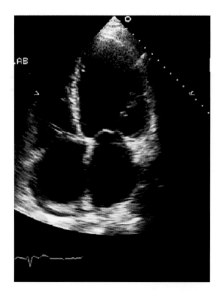

A. Ebstein's anomaly
B. Hypertrophic cardiomyopathy
C. Atrial septal defect (ASD)
D. Dilated cardiomyopathy

3. The most likely mechanism of mitral regurgitation (MR) in this patient is:

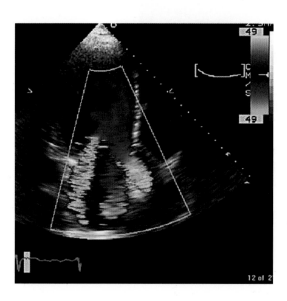

A. P2 tethering
B. P2 prolapse
C. Bileaflet mitral valve prolapse
D. None of the above

4. This 19-year-old patient was stabbed in the precordial area. Examination revealed a loud systolic murmur. The most likely cause of this murmur is:

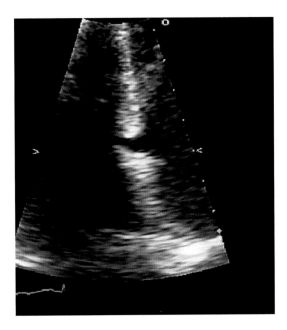

A. Penetrating injury to the interventricular septum
B. Mitral valve prolapse
C. Hypertrophic obstructive cardiomyopathy (HOCM)
D. None of the above

5. This transesophageal echocardiogram (TEE) image is obtained from the upper esophagus, and the aortic arch is shown on the top. The arrow points to:

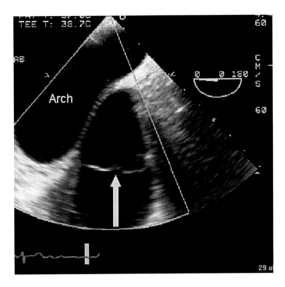

A. Pulmonary valve
B. Aortic valve
C. Mitral valve
D. Tricuspid valve

6. The structure indicated by the arrow is:

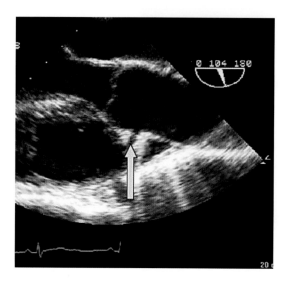

A. Right coronary artery (RCA)
B. Left coronary artery (LCA)
C. Entry tear into dissection
D. None of the above

7. This is a suprasternal image of the aortic arch, suggestive of:

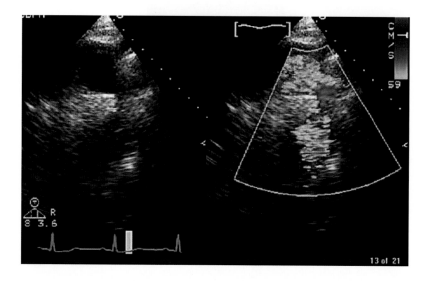

A. Coarctation of the aorta
B. Severe aortic regurgitation (AR)
C. Patent ductus arteriosus (PDA)
D. None of the above

8. The structure indicated by the arrow is:

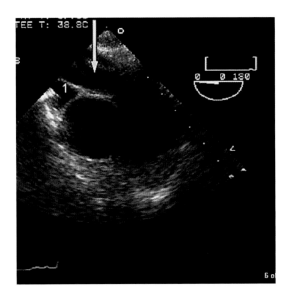

A. Right pulmonary artery (RPA)
B. Left atrium
C. Aortic arch
D. Right upper pulmonary vein

9. The structure denoted by the arrow is:

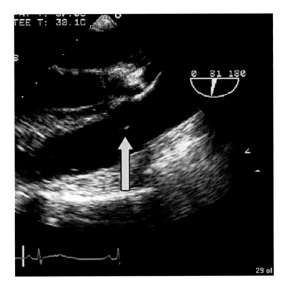

A. Artifact
B. Pulmonary valve
C. Aortic valve
D. Subpulmonic stenosis

10. The abnormality in this image is:

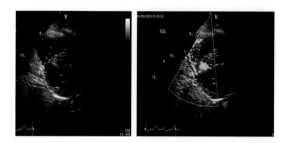

A. Congenital muscular ventricular septal defect (VSD)
B. Postinfarction posterior VSD
C. Artifact of the normal posterior thinning at the valve plane
D. Postmyectomy of HOCM

11. The abnormal finding in this image is:

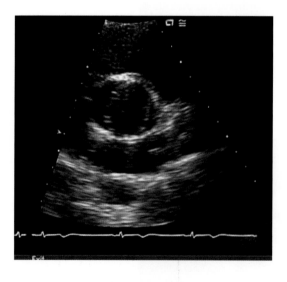

A. Bicuspid aortic valve
B. Aortic dissection flap
C. Aortic aneurysm
D. None of the above

12. The MR signal shown here is suggestive of:

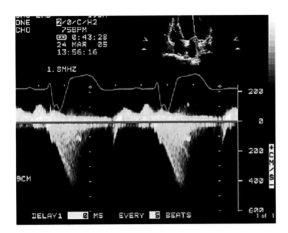

A. Some diastolic MR in addition to systolic MR
B. Markedly depressed left ventricular (LV) dp/dt
C. Both of the above
D. Neither of the above

13. The mitral flow profile shown here is suggestive of:

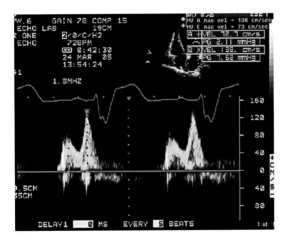

A. Normal LV diastolic function
B. Abnormal relaxation
C. Pseudonormal pattern
D. Restrictive pattern

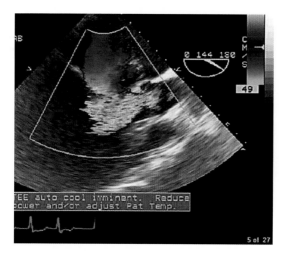

A. Normal flow in the left ventricular outflow tract (LVOT)
B. Subvalvular aortic stenosis (AS)
C. AR
D. None of the above

15. This continuous wave Doppler signal is suggestive of:

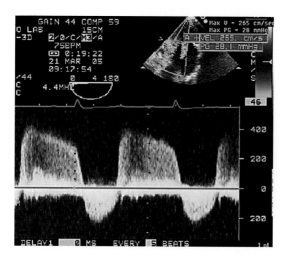

A. AS and AR
B. Mitral stenosis (MS) and MR
C. VSD flow
D. Aortic flow in a patient with coarctation

16. This continuous wave signal obtained from the mid-transesophageal location is indicative of:

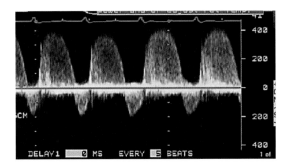

A. AS and AR
B. MS and MR
C. VSD flow
D. None of the above

17. This is a TEE image from the mid-esophagus of a late diastolic frame of the aortic valve. This patient is most likely to have:

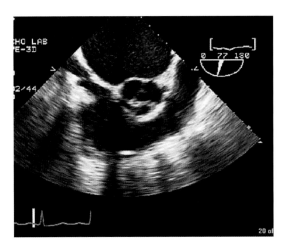

A. Severe AR
B. Severe AS
C. HOCM
D. Ascending aortic dissection

18. This patient is most likely to have:

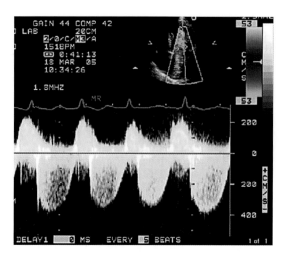

   A. Acute severe MR
   B. Chronic severe MR
   C. Severe MS and mild MR
   D. None of the above

19. This patient had *Staphylococcus aureus* endocarditis of the aortic valve. The most likely cause is:

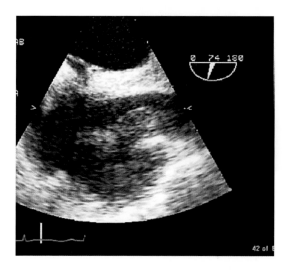

   A. Central venous catheter-associated infection
   B. Dental work
   C. Immunosuppressed state
   D. Intravenous drug use

20. The image of the aortic valve is suggestive of:

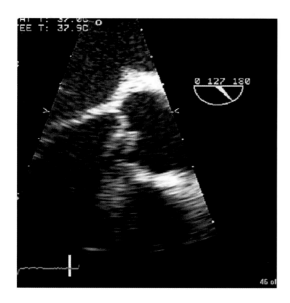

A. Aortic valve vegetation
B. Node of Arantius
C. Lambl's excrescences
D. Ascending aortic dissection causing prolapse of the noncoronary cusp

Answers for Chapter 17

1. **Answer: A.**
   Left heart failure. The mitral inflow shown here is indicative of high left atrial (LA) pressure. Although the patient is in atrial fibrillation with only E-wave, the E-wave deceleration is very rapid, with a deceleration time of 100 ms.

2. **Answer: D.**
   Dilated cardiomyopathy. There is a four-chamber dilatation. There is no increase in wall thickness to suggest HOCM. In ASD both the right ventricle and the right atrium will be dilated due to volume overload with normal LA and LV size. The tricuspid valve position is normal and hence does not support the diagnosis of Ebstein's anomaly.

3. **Answer: A.**
   P2 tethering. This is an apical long axis view, showing A2 and P2 scallops of the mitral valve. The MR jet is directed posterolaterally toward P2, consistent with P2 tethering. A similar jet direction can also occur in A2 prolapse, but both leaflets coapt distal to the plane of mitral annulus. Bileaflet prolapse of equal magnitude will result in a central jet.

4. **Answer: A.**
   Penetrating injury to the interventricular septum. A defect is seen in the ventricular septum. This patient had a penetrating injury to the septum. The image does not support the presence of mitral valve prolapse or hypertrophic septum.

5. **Answer: A.**
   Pulmonary valve. Pulmonary valve and the main pulmonary artery are seen. This is a good view to examine these structures and also to obtain spectral Doppler signals from the pulmonary valve and pulmonary artery. The main pulmonary artery is closer to the transducer.

6. **Answer: A.**
   This is the classical location of the RCA. The LCA is not seen in the aortic long axis view. Because of its left lateral location, it is seen in the short axis view. There is no aortic dissection and entry tear into dissection would be a hole in the endothelium and is not tubular in shape.

7. **Answer: A.**
   Coarctation of the aorta. Narrowing and turbulence at the junction of the arch and descending aorta are clearly seen, indicative of coarctation. In severe AR, flow reversal is holodiastolic. This is a systolic frame (see marker on the ECG). There is no communication between the aorta and the pulmonary artery, suggestive of PDA.

8. **Answer: A.**
   RPA. This is a TEE image from the proximal esophageal location, a high basal view above the level of the left atrium. Also note the linear shadows in the RPA, which are commonly seen and represent mirror image artifacts. A short axis image of the RPA or color flow image at a low scale would confirm this. The large circular structure is the ascending aorta and number 1 is the SVC in cross-section. Also note the reverberations from a catheter in the SVC.

9. **Answer: B.**

Pulmonary valve. This is a TEE image from mid to low esophageal location showing the long axis of the pulmonary valve and the proximal pulmonary artery. The right ventricular outflow tract is clearly seen as well.

10. **Answer: B.**

Postinfarction posterior VSD. There is marked thinning of the mid-inferior wall and inferior septum without any scarring. There is also a defect establishing communication between the LV and the RV and the color flow confirms this. This is classical postinfarct posterior VSD, and a short axis view of the LV at all levels would help to delineate the pathology. Such thinning does not occur in congenital VSD. The location of iatrogenic infarct or myectomy in HOCM is in the proximal anterior septum.

11. **Answer: A.**

This is a classic bicuspid aortic valve. Although a dissection flap in a patient with circumferential dissection with a central true lumen may mimic this, both leaflets and commissures are clearly seen here. This image is at the level of the aortic annulus and the rest of the ascending aorta is not shown to comment about nondissecting aortic aneurysm.

12. **Answer: C.**

Both. The initial portion of the signal at low velocity represents diastolic MR, which occurs during LA relaxation and may be due to a long PR interval or high left ventricular end diastolic pressure (LVEDP). The rate of velocity rise of the MR signal is very slow. The normal time taken for the MR velocity to increase from 1 to 3 m/s is 10–20 ms, representing an LV dp/dt of 1600–3200 mmHg/s. In this example this interval is 160 ms, giving an average rate of pressure rise during early systole (loosely called LV dp/dt and correlating with this) is 200 mmHg/s. Also note the very prolonged QRS duration. The main determinants of LV dp/dt include LV contractility, heart rate, preload, and LV systolic synchrony, which would be abnormal in left bundle branch block.

13. **Answer: B.**

Abnormal relaxation, suggested by an E/A ratio of < 1. Although the E-wave deceleration time is < 250 ms, generally the isovolumic relaxation time (not shown here) tends to be greater than 100 ms. The E/A ratio can be lower in the elderly because of age-related LV relaxation failure, patients with low filling pressures, more rapid heart rates, and those with prolongation of the PR interval. In a pseudonormal pattern the mitral inflow looks normal, but there is some other evidence of LV relaxation abnormality, such as reduced Em velocity, reduced mitral flow propagation, or increased duration of atrial systole as judged by pulmonary vein flow (AR-wave reversal duration). Restrictive pattern is characterized by an E/A ratio of > 2, E-wave deceleration of < 150 ms, and isovolumic relaxation time of < 70 ms.

14. **Answer: C.**

AR. Note the diastolic frame showing an AR jet. The AR is severe as the width of the jet is > 60% of the LVOT and has a large vena contracta and proximal isovelocity surface area (PISA).

15. **Answer: A.**

AS and AR. Unlike the MR signal, the AS signal occupies only the ejection period and is absent during the isovolumic contraction time. Hence, the signal starts a few milliseconds after the QRS. The diastolic velocity is too high for MS. This order of gradient and LA pressure would be incompatible with life. VSD flow is predominantly systolic with a presystolic component caused by atrial contraction. The gradient across a coarctation is systolic, the duration increases with greater degrees of stenosis, and there may be a diastolic gradient. However, both the systolic and diastolic components will be in the same direction.

16. **Answer: B.**
MS and MR. See the explanation to Question 335. Note that in TEE from a mid-esophageal location, the MR jet is directed toward the transducer.

17. **Answer: A.**
Severe AR. The aortic leaflets are thickened with rolled-up edges and a central coaptation defect in end diastole. This anatomy would be associated with wide-open AR, as the regurgitant orifice is visible by anatomic imaging. AS cannot be diagnosed by a diastolic frame. HOCM typically causes midsystolic closure of the aortic valve, best visualized by M mode. Aortic dissection may cause AR by one of several mechanisms: dilatation of sino-tubular junction, leaflet tethering, extension of hematoma into the aortic leaflet causing it to prolapse, or as a result of the primary problem such as bicuspid aortic valve or annulo-aortic ectasia.

18. **Answer: B.**
Chronic severe MR. The MR signal density is more than 60% of the mitral inflow signal. This correlates with a volume of regurgitation. In addition, the mitral inflow velocity is increased without a slow deceleration. A slow deceleration would indicate significant MS. Despite severe MR, the profile of the MR signal is quite rounded, without the rapid deceleration that would typically be seen in acute severe MR, because of the large LA V-wave, the so-called V-wave cutoff sign. Note that the heart rate is 151 beats/min. At rapid heart rates MR may be grossly underestimated by color Doppler due to limited temporal resolution and continuous wave Doppler is very helpful.

19. **Answer: A.**
Central venous catheter-associated infection. This bicaval transesophageal view shows a large mass in the SVC, which is typically associated with a central catheter-associated thrombus or vegetation. This most likely is the cause of his sepsis and endocarditis. In addition, there is a possible defect at the superior portion of the fossa ovalis, suggesting a patent foramen ovale (PFO). This patient had a large PFO by color and contrast echocardiography, allowing paradoxical embolization of the bacterial mass to cause left-sided endocarditis, escaping the protective filtration mechanism offered by the lung.

20. **Answer: A.**
Aortic valve vegetation. The mass on the aortic valve is suggestive of a mass on the LV side of the aortic valve. This is suggestive of vegetation. Also, there is pro-lapse of the noncoronary cusp, causing significant AR, and this is due to leaflet destruction with endocarditis. The other mechanism for prolapse could be a bicuspid aortic valve with prolapse of the larger cusp. The node of Arantius, as the name suggests, is a nodular thickening of the central portion of the leaflet edge and is best visualized from the short axis view of the valve. Lambl's excrescences are thin filamentous structures attached to the leaflet margin. There is no evidence of aortic dissection or intramural hematoma in this patient.

18

Questions

1. This continuous wave Doppler signal is indicative of:

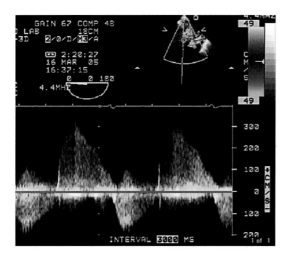

A. Acute severe aortic regurgitation (AR)
B. Chronic compensated AR
C. Severe aortic stenosis (AS)
D. Severe mixed mitral valve disease

Echocardiography Board Review: 600 Multiple Choice Questions with Discussion, Third Edition.
Ramdas G. Pai and Padmini Varadarajan.
© 2025 John Wiley & Sons Ltd. Published 2025 by John Wiley & Sons Ltd.

2. This transesophageal echocardiogram (TEE) image is suggestive of:

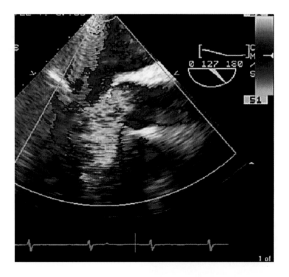

    A. Severe AR
    B. Hypertrophic obstructive cardiomyopathy (HOCM)
    C. Subaortic membranous AS
    D. None of the above

3. This pulse wave Doppler flow signal in the descending thoracic aorta on a TEE is indicative of:

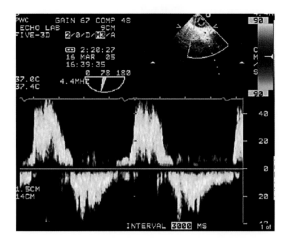

    A. Coarctation of the aorta
    B. Middle aortic syndrome

C. Severe AR

D. HOCM

4. What procedure did this patient undergo?

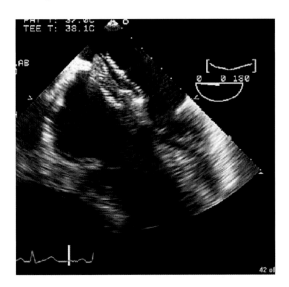

A. Mitral valve replacement

B. Atrial septal defect (ASD) closure with an Amplatzer device

C. Patent foramen ovale (PFO) closure with a cardioseal device

D. ASD closure with a pericardial patch

5. This patient is likely to have:

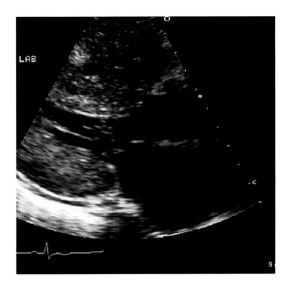

A. Systolic murmur accentuated by Valsalva maneuver
B. Early peaking systolic murmur
C. Early diastolic murmur heard in sitting position at end expiration
D. A mid-diastolic murmur best heard with the bell in left lateral position

6. This signal shown here is likely to be caused by:

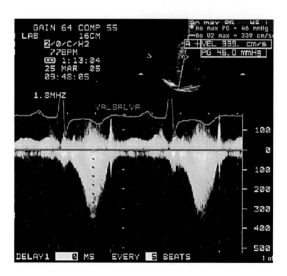

A. HOCM
B. Critical valvular AS
C. Acute mitral regurgitation (MR)
D. None of the above

7. The image shown here is suggestive of:

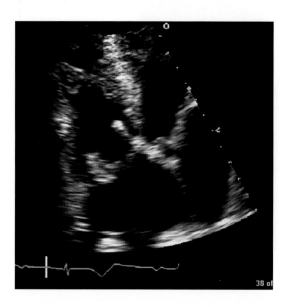

A. Bioprosthetic tricuspid valve
B. Carcinoid valvulopathy of the tricuspid valve
C. Tricuspid annuloplasty ring
D. Large tricuspid vegetation

8. This 65-year-old patient with MR is likely to have:

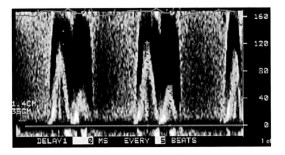

A. An opening snap
B. Third heart sound
C. Fourth heart sound
D. Summation gallop

9. The continuous wave Doppler signal is consistent with:

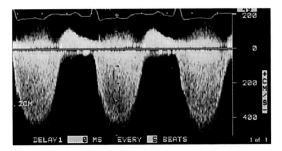

A. Critical AS
B. Severe MR
C. Maladie de Roger
D. None of the above

10. This tricuspid regurgitation (TR) signal was obtained from TEE. The clinically estimated right atrial (RA) pressure in this patient was 20 mmHg and there is no pulmonary stenosis. The pulmonary artery (PA) systolic pressure in this patient would be:

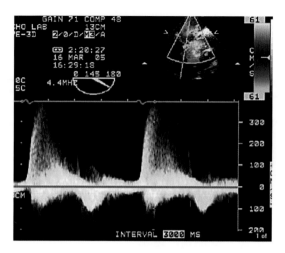

A. 30 mmHg
B. 50 mmHg
C. 80 mmHg
D. Cannot be calculated

11. This patient is likely to have:

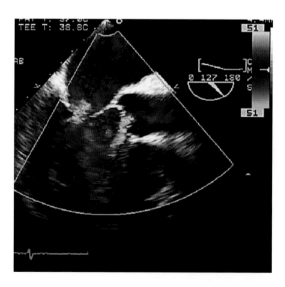

A. Acute severe AR
B. Mild AR
C. Mitral stenosis
D. None of the above

12. This transmitral flow is obtained from the esophageal transducer location from a patient with *Staphylococcus aureus* bacteremia and acute hemodynamic

decompensation. The patient is in sinus rhythm. The most likely cause of his decompensation is:

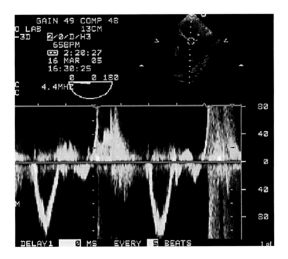

  A. Acute MR
  B. Acute AR
  C. Rupture of the ventricular septum
  D. None of the above

13. The cause of this patient's multiple bilateral lung abscesses is:

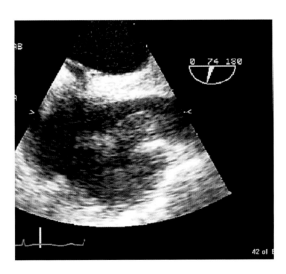

  A. Vegetation in the superior vena cava (SVC)
  B. Tricuspid endocarditis
  C. Probable immune deficiency; no vegetation seen on the image
  D. None of the above

14. The cause of heart failure in this 30-year-old man is likely to be:

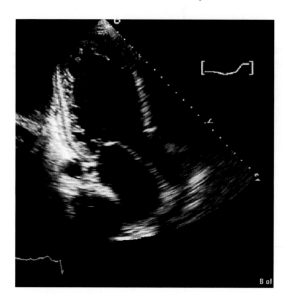

   A. Noncompaction of the left ventricle (LV)
   B. Hemochromatosis
   C. Cardiac amyloid
   D. Hypertrophic cardiomyopathy

15. The structure indicated by the arrow is:

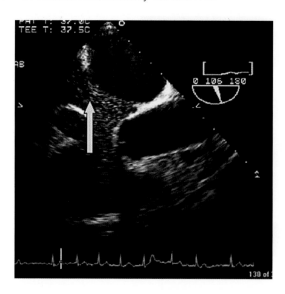

   A. Inferior vena cava (IVC)– RA junction
   B. SVC
   C. Anomalously draining right upper pulmonary vein
   D. ASD

16. The MR flow rate in this patient – proximal isovelocity surface area (PISA) radius of 0.9 cm, aliasing velocity of 38 cm/s – is approximately:

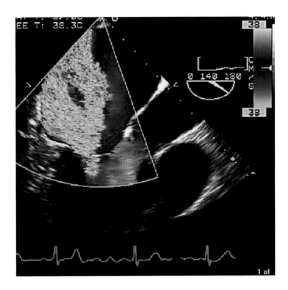

A. 200 cc/s
B. 200 cc/min
C. 100 cc/min
D. 100 cc/s

17. The patient shown is likely to have:

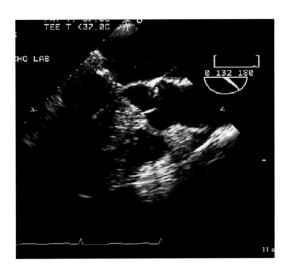

A. Early diastolic murmur
B. Late peaking systolic ejection murmur with absence of A2 component of S2
C. Late peaking systolic murmur increased by Valsalva's maneuver and normal A2
D. Mid-diastolic murmur

18. The most likely diagnosis in this patient is:

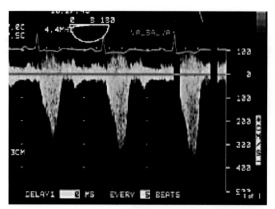

At rest

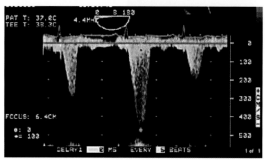

With Valsalva

A. HOCM
B. Severe AS
C. Mitral valve prolapse
D. None of the above

19. This patient is likely to have:

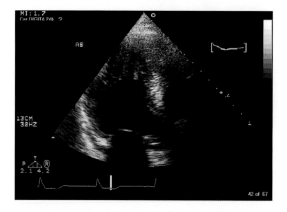

A. Apical HOCM
B. Hypertensive heart disease
C. Endomyocardial fibrosis
D. None of the above

20. The appearance of the atrial septum in this patient is due to:

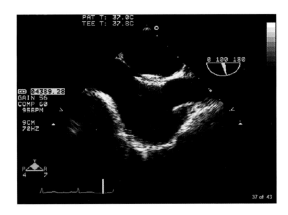

A. ASD repair with a pericardial patch
B. ASD closure device
C. PFO closure device
D. None of the above

Answers for Chapter 18

1. **Answer: A.**
   Acute severe AR. There is a rapid deceleration of the AR velocity profile indicating rapidly diminishing aorto–left ventricular (LV) pressure gradient, which is typically seen in acute severe AR, mostly due to rapid rise in LV diastolic pressure, due to regurgitation in a noncompliant nonconditioned left ventricle. It is also possible to get this in chronic severe AR with severe vasodilatation, which would cause a low aortic diastolic pressure, but this scenario is less frequent. The systolic signal is early peaking, with a velocity of only 2 m/s, and severe AR indicating the absence of any significant AS. The onset of the systolic signal after the isovolumic contraction period indicates its origin at the semilunar valve as opposed to an origin at the A–V valve. This systolic velocity is too low for MR unless the continuous wave signal is malaligned to the MR jet direction; this is unlikely as the signal is not bidirectional and the diastolic velocity is too high for MS.

2. **Answer: A.**
   Severe AR. This diastolic frame is indicated by the open mitral valve, and the left ventricular outflow tract (LVOT) is completely filled with turbulent flow typical of wide-open AR. Note that this is not a systolic frame to indicate subvalvular AS.

3. **Answer: C.**
   Severe AR. A prominent holodiastolic flow reversal suggesting retrograde flow in the aorta is seen. This flow would also cause Duroziez's murmur by physical exam due to the turbulence produced by partial occlusion by the finger, which would produce a diastolic murmur in the proximal femoral artery. Coarctation and middle aortic syndrome diminish pulsatility in the distal aortic flow and the flow becomes continuous due to flow through collaterals. Although HOCM can produce mid-systolic closure of the aortic valve, it does not produce any flow disturbance in the distal aorta.

4. **Answer: B.**
   ASD closure with Amplatzer. This is a typical appearance of an Amplatzer device. Both the left and RA disks are seen, sandwiching the atrial septum. The role of TEE during ASD closure includes sizing of the defect, with and without balloon inflation, examination of adequacy of rims, ruling out anomalous pulmonary venous connections, guiding deployment, and ascertaining post-deployment lack of impingement into SVC, right upper pulmonary vein, IVC, and the mitral valve, in addition to excluding any residual ASD. Small flow through the device is normal until it becomes endothelialized.

5. **Answer: A.**
   Systolic murmur accentuated by Valsalva's maneuver. This is a mid-systolic frame showing systolic anterior motion (SAM) of the anterior mitral leaflet. As SAM increases in late systole, the gradient will be maximal in end systole, causing a late peaking systolic murmur. Both the gradient and murmur are increased by Valsalva's maneuver through a diminution of LV volume, causing an increase in SAM. Early diastolic murmur heard in the sitting position at end expiration is typical of AR. A mid-diastolic murmur best heard with the bell in the left lateral position is typical of mitral stenosis.

6. **Answer: A.**

   HOCM. This late peaking dagger-shaped signal is typical of SAM caused by HOCM. This occurs due to the dynamic LVOT obstruction increases through systole. Critical valvular AS is unlikely, as in this case the velocity is likely to be higher (unless cardiac output is very low) and the signal contour would be more rounded. Acute MR gives rise to an early peaking signal with a rapid deceleration because of a large left atrial (LA) V-wave, the so-called V-wave cut-off sign. In LV cavity obliteration this signal will be much later peaking, with a gradient only in the very late part of systole when there is very little blood left in the distal LV cavity.

7. **Answer: A.**

   Bioprosthetic tricuspid valve. This patient has a Hancock porcine bioprosthetic tricuspid valve. The struts of the bioprosthetic valve are easily seen. An annuloplasty ring would be seen as a small rounded structure in cross-section at the tricuspid annulus only.

8. **Answer: B.**

   Third heart sound. The mitral inflow is suggestive of high LA pressure. The mitral E/A ratio is > 2 and deceleration time is 60 ms, indicating very high LA pressure. The E-wave deceleration calculated from the E-wave amplitude and its time (velocity/time) is about $20\,m/s^2$. A rate of deceleration of > 8–$9\,m/s^2$ is likely to result in S3. Age is relevant, as such a filling pattern in young children is normal because they have extremely efficient LV relaxation, which would result in physiological S3. S4 results from a prominent atrial filling wave in a stiff ventricle, and in a summation gallop the E- and A-waves are fused. This patient has no mitral stenosis and hence opening snap is unlikely.

9. **Answer: B.**

   Severe MR. The temporal continuity of the systolic signal with the inflow signal suggests its origin at the mitral valve. The AS signal would occupy only the ejection period, being separated from the mitral inflow signal by isovolumic contraction and relaxation periods. A small ventricular septal defect (VSD) may result in a holosystolic signal but generally has a presystolic component associated LA systole, and usually this flow is directed toward the transducer from most of the imaging windows.

10. **Answer: C.**

    80 mmHg. The TR velocity is 4 m/s, yielding an right ventricular (RV)–RA systolic gradient of 64 mmHg. With an RA pressure of 20 mmHg, the RV systolic pressure would be about 80 mmHg, which would be the same as the PA systolic pressure in the absence of significant pulmonic stenosis.

11. **Answer: A.**

    Acute severe AR. This late diastolic frame shows diastolic MR. There is also AR by color. The mitral valve is closed prematurely. This combination of findings is consistent with acute severe AR. A smaller AR jet in late diastole was because of late diastolic equilibration of aortic and left ventricular pressures. Diastolic MR results from the receipt of AR volume in an LV with high operating end diastolic stiffness.

12. **Answer: B.**

    Acute AR. The Doppler flow suggests premature closure of the mitral valve with lack of A-wave despite being in sinus rhythm. This is pathognomonic of acute AR causing rapidly rising LV diastolic pressure due to failure to accommodate a large acute volume overload. In acute AR, the LA would still be contracting but would be unable to eject against an acute increase in afterload. Pulmonary vein flow profile in this patient would show a prominent AR wave and the tricuspid inflow would still have the A-wave. Acute MR and VSD would not eliminate the A-wave unless the patient had a recent episode of atrial fibrillation and the atrium is stunned.

13. **Answer: A.**
    Vegetation in SVC. The image shows large vegetation protruding into the right atrium. This was catheter related causing *Staphylococcus* bacteremia. Imaging the whole length of the SVC, RA endocardium, and the Eustachian valve is extremely important in patients with central catheters or peripherally inserted central catheter (PICC) lines with fever or suspected bacteremia.

14. **Answer: A.**
    Noncompaction of the LV. The inferolateral wall of the LV in this patient is heavily trabeculated; noncompacted (trabeculated) to compacted wall thickness ratio is more than 2:1. This is highly indicative of noncompaction of LV myocardium, which is a developmental disorder causing congestive heart failure. In the other three conditions the LV myocardium would be thicker, either due to infiltration or increased myocardial mass.

15. **Answer: A.**
    IVC–right atrium junction. Part of the proximal IVC is seen with entry of saline contrast in the longitudinal plane from a TEE. With this orientation caudal structures are seen on the left and cephalad structures are seen on the right. This patient has a prominent Eustachian valve, and in a patient with a prominent Eustachian valve in a low esophageal view, where the LA is not seen, this junction may be mistaken for an ASD. This patient was referred from an outside facility with that mistaken diagnosis from a TEE.

16. **Answer: A.**
    200 cc/s. The regurgitant flow rate equals $2\pi r2 \times$ Nyquist limit. Here, the PISA radius is 0.9 cm and the Nyquist limit is 38 cm/s. Regurgitant flow rate = $6.28 \times 0.9 \times 0.9 \times 38 = 200$ cc/s.

17. **Answer: C.**
    This patient clearly has SAM of the anterior mitral leaflet causing LVOT obstruction. As the SAM increases in late systole, the gradient velocity and turbulence are more in late systole, causing a late peaking late systolic murmur. SAM is increased by LV volume reduction and vasodilatation. A2 is preserved in these patients in contrast to patients with severe AS, who may also have late peaking systolic murmur.

18. **Answer: A.**
    HOCM. This patient has HOCM with dynamic LVOT obstruction caused by SAM, which causes a late peaking systolic gradient, increased by Valsalva's maneuver and amyl nitrate inhalation. The gradient would also be increased by positive inotropic agents and vasodilators and decreased by an increase in afterload, with vasoconstrictors or handgrip. In addition to HOCM, SAM can occur in volume-depleted states with small LV cavity and also after surgical mitral valve repair in patients with long anterior and posterior leaflets, especially if a small annuloplasty ring is used.

19. **Answer: A.**

Apical HOCM. This patient has disproportionately thickened LV apical myocardium typical of apical HOCM. This results in a spade-shaped LV cavity in diastole. These patients also have giant T-wave inversions in their chest leads. In hypertensive heart disease LV hypotension is more uniformly distributed. Endomyocardial fibrosis causes apical obliteration due to endocardial thickening rather than myocardial thickening.

20. **Answer: C.**

PFO closure device. The image shows two parallel disks sandwiching the upper atrial septum. The RA disk is larger than the LA disk. This is suggestive of an Amplatzer PFO closure device. In an ASD closure device, the LA disk is larger than the RA disk. Patch repair of the septum will not show the triple-layer morphology as seen here.

19

Questions

1. The image shows:

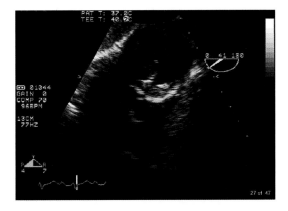

   A. Normal native tricuspid valve
   B. Normal bioprosthetic valve
   C. Vegetation on a bioprosthetic valve
   D. Avulsion of the tricuspid valve

2. This 31-year-old woman with no other medical history had two episodes of transient ischemic cerebral attacks, the first one after a long duration of air travel and the second one during straining in the restroom. The most likely cause of this patient's attacks is:

Echocardiography Board Review: 600 Multiple Choice Questions with Discussion, Third Edition.
Ramdas G. Pai and Padmini Varadarajan.
© 2025 John Wiley & Sons Ltd. Published 2025 by John Wiley & Sons Ltd.

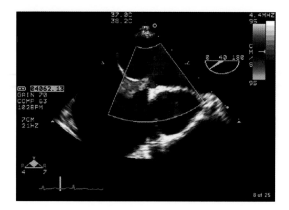

A. Paradoxical embolism
B. Vagally mediated atrial fibrillation
C. Left atrial thrombus
D. None of the above

3. This 35-year-old patient with AIDS and bicuspid aortic valve has *Staphylococcus* bacteremia. The parasternal long axis color flow image is suggestive of:

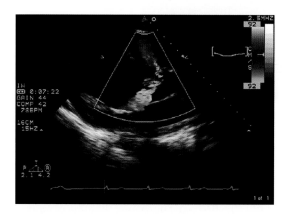

A. Right coronary artery flow
B. Pulmonary vegetation
C. Fistulous communication between aorta and right ventricle (RV)
D. None of the above

4. This patient's bilateral *Staphylococcus* lung abscesses are likely due to:

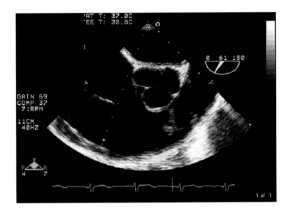

    A. Tricuspid valve endocarditis
    B. Pulmonary valve endocarditis
    C. Catheter-related infection of superior vena cava and right atrium (RA)
    D. None of the above

5. The structure indicated by the arrow is:

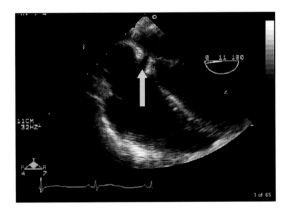

    A. Coronary sinus
    B. Inferior vena cava
    C. Atrial septal defect
    D. None of the above

6. This patient's stroke is likely due to:

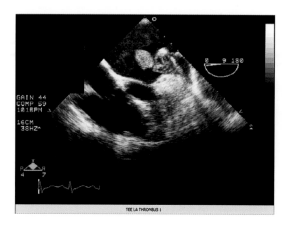

A. Left atrial thrombus
B. Left atrial myxoma
C. Mitral valve endocarditis
D. Patent foramen ovale (PFO)

7. The structure indicated by the arrow is:

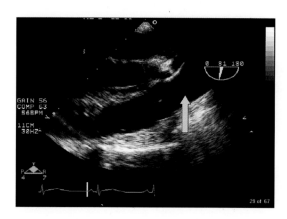

A. Main pulmonary artery (PA)
B. Ascending aorta
C. Descending aorta
D. None of the above

8. This patient with a prosthetic tricuspid valve has evidence of:

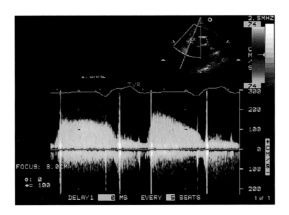

- A. Normal function
- B. Stenosis
- C. Regurgitation
- D. Endocarditis

9. The mass in the left atrium in this patient is most likely:

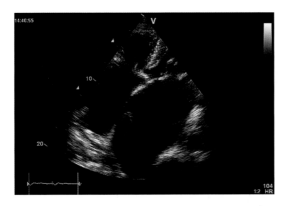

- A. Thrombus
- B. Myxoma
- C. Metastatic lung carcinoma
- D. Lipomatous septum

10. The short axis view of the heart is indicative of:

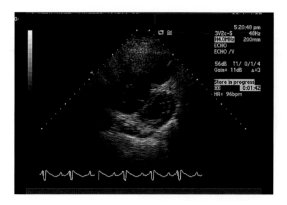

    A. Severe pulmonary hypertension
    B. Severe tricuspid regurgitation (TR) with normal PA pressure
    C. RV infarct
    D. RV dysplasia

11. The surgical procedure that this patient underwent is most likely to be:

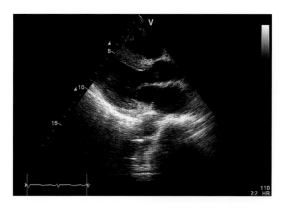

    A. Orthotropic heart transplantation
    B. Mitral valve repair with annuloplasty
    C. Maze procedure
    D. Septal myectomy for hypertrophic obstructive cardiomyopathy

12. This TR signal is from a patient with moderate TR. The most likely mechanism of TR is:

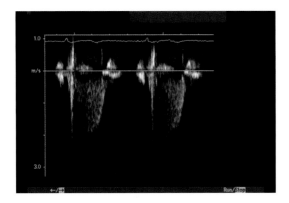

A. Pulmonary hypertension with annular dilatation
B. Flail tricuspid valve
C. Tricuspid valve prolapse
D. Cannot make a mechanistic diagnosis

13. This image of the aortic arch from the suprasternal view is suggestive of:

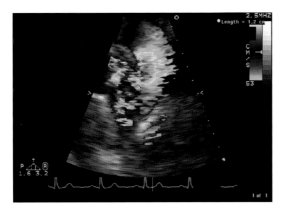

A. Patent ductus arteriosus (PDA)
B. Coarctation of the aorta
C. Severe aortic regurgitation
D. Aortic pseudoaneurysm

14. A 42-year-old woman presented with complaints of shortness of breath. An echocardiogram was obtained. Dynamic images showed an LV ejection fraction of 50% with abnormal appearance of the apex. Filling pressures were high, valves

were normal. She had a normal electrocardiogram and a comprehensive and complete blood count except an eosinophil count of 20%. The appearance of the LV apex is suggestive of:

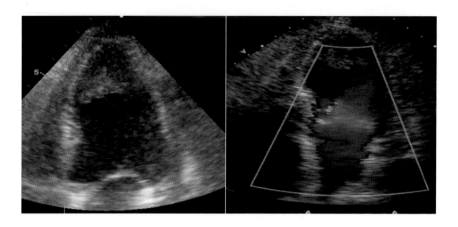

A. LV apical thrombus
B. LV noncompaction
C. Apical hypertrophic cardiomyopathy
D. Endomyocardial fibrosis

15. The TR velocity profile shown here is suggestive of:

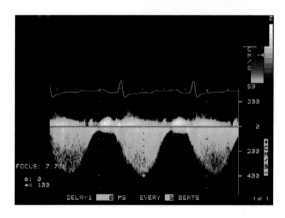

A. Normal PA pressure
B. Mild pulmonary hypertension
C. Severe pulmonary hypertension with good RV function
D. Severe pulmonary hypertension with poor RV function

16. The amount of TR in this patient is:

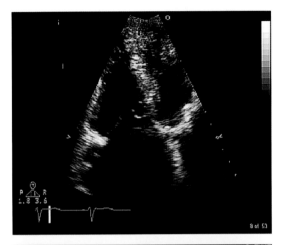

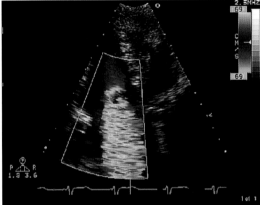

A. Mild
B. Moderate
C. Severe
D. Cannot quantify

17. The patient in Question 16 is likely to have:

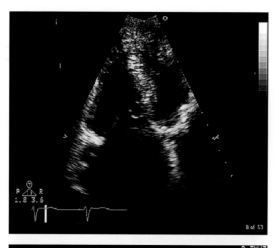

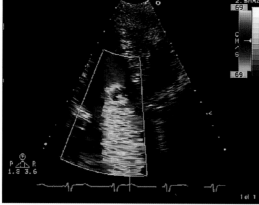

A. Normal PA pressure
B. Mild pulmonary hypertension
C. Moderate or severe pulmonary hypertension

18. The type of surgical procedure performed on this patient's mitral valve is likely to be:

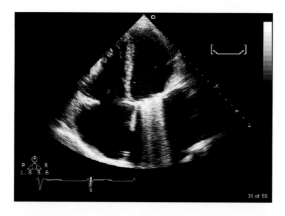

A. Mitral annuloplasty
B. Alfieri procedure
C. Replacement with a bioprosthetic valve
D. Replacement with a mechanical valve

19. What intervention can potentially change the mitral inflow pattern as shown in this image?

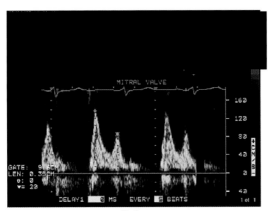

Before

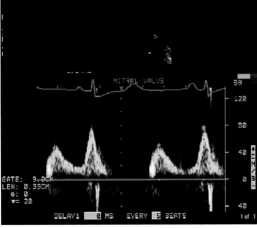

After

A. Diuresis
B. Control of severe hypertension
C. Correction of severe anemia
D. All of the above

20. The abnormality shown in this image is:

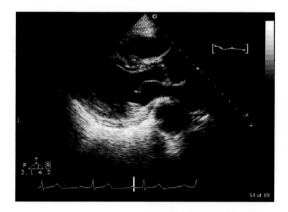

A. Thoracic aortic aneurysm
B. Cor triatriatum
C. Artifact
D. Dilated left PA

Answers for Chapter 19

1. **Answer: C.**
   Vegetation on a bioprosthetic valve. This is a short axis view of the tricuspid valve, best obtained from a proximal gastric location, with clockwise probe rotation at about 20–30 degrees. The sewing ring of the prosthetic valve is clearly seen here and there is a mass attached to the leaflets indicative of vegetation.

2. **Answer: A.**
   Paradoxical embolism. The transesophageal echocardiogram image shows the interatrial septum with a large PFO in its typical location. The color flow shows left to right flow. This flow would reverse under situations of increased RA pressure such as straining, coughing, and right heart failure. The orientation of the opening is favorable for thrombi originating in the inferior vena cava region to traverse the PFO to the left atrium even in the absence of raised RA pressure.

3. **Answer: C.**
   Fistulous communication between the aorta and the RV. In addition to the fistulous communication, the image also shows aortic regurgitation. Fistulous communications generally result from rupture of an aortic root abscess. This may result in communications to the RA, RV, PA, or the left ventricular outflow tract (LVOT). Other local complications include abscess of mitral aortic intervalvular fibrosa, leaflet aneurysm, and perforation of the anterior mitral leaflet. One may also get an abscess in the ventricular septum, causing a ventricular septal defect after rupture.

4. **Answer: B.**
   Pulmonary valve endocarditis. This is a mid-esophageal image showing the aortic valve in short axis in the center and the RV inflow and outflow wrapped around it akin to the short axis of the aortic valve from a parasternal view. There is a large mass attached to the pulmonary valve consistent with vegetation. This is the likely source of his lung abscesses.

5. **Answer: A.**
   Coronary sinus. This is a low esophageal view partially cutting through the posterior A–V groove showing the coronary sinus.

6. **Answer: A.**
   Left atrial thrombus. This patient has a large left atrium with spontaneous echocontrast, with large masses originating from the left atrial appendage suggestive of thrombi. These are protruding into the body of the left atrium. These masses were highly mobile and the patient had rheumatic mitral stenosis, although the mitral valve is not visualized here. Note that this patient is in sinus rhythm. In patients with mitral stenosis, thrombi can form despite being in sinus rhythm because of stasis in a large atrium, another possible mechanism being paroxysmal atrial fibrillation. Myxoma generally arises from the atrial septum, and mitral vegetations generally arise from the atrial side of the leaflets and usually do not grow to such a massive size.

7. **Answer: A.**
   Main PA. This view is obtained from the mid-esophageal view, with anterior structures displayed away from the transducer and superior structures to the right. This is a typical tomographic view showing right ventricular outflow tract,

pulmonary valve, and main PA. Part of the LVOT and aortic valve is seen posterior to this. Pulling the probe up slightly will show the distal PA and proximal branches can be seen from a much more proximal location in the esophagus from a horizontal plane.

8. **Answer: B.**
Stenosis. This is suggested by the increased transvalvular velocity associated with a slow deceleration time. The peak diastolic gradient is 16 mmHg, mean gradient is 8 mmHg, and the pressure half-time is markedly prolonged at 250–300 ms, suggesting severe tricuspid stenosis. The pressure half-time method is not validated for calculating the effective orifice area of either native or prosthetic tricuspid valves. Generally a mean transvalvular gradient of > 5 mmHg is suggestive of severe tricuspid stenosis. As the gradient is flow dependent, it varies with the phase of respiration.

9. **Answer: A.**
Thrombus. The differential diagnosis is between thrombus and left atrial myxoma. In this patient with a giant left atrium, who is likely to be in atrial fibrillation, this is more likely to be a thrombus. The fact that the mass is not pedunculated and has a homogenous acoustic characteristic favors a diagnosis of thrombus, although the possibility of myxoma cannot be excluded. If vascularity is shown in the mass by color flow imaging or contrast echocardiography with transpulmonary agents, then it would suggest myxoma. Lipomatous septum is dumbbell-shaped with sparing of the fossa ovalis. Lung carcinoma propagates to the left atrium through pulmonary veins and the mass generally originates in one of the pulmonary veins.

10. **Answer: A.**
Severe pulmonary hypertension. Note that this is a systolic frame and the interventricular septum is flattened, indicating an RV pressure closer or equal to the LV pressure. The ventricular septum responds passively to the transmural pressure and hence generally is convex to RV both in systole and diastole because of the higher LV pressure. Severe TR with normal PA pressure would cause diastolic flattening of the septum, and the septum would be rounded in systole as the LV pressure is higher. In RV dysplasia, RV is dilated, thin walled with occasional aneurysms, and the septum would be flattened in diastole. In RV infarct, PA pressure would be normal.

11. **Answer: A.**
Orthotropic heart transplantation. The ridge-like projection seen on the posterior left atrial wall is the site of anastomosis between donor and recipient left atria. The pulmonary venous side of the atria belongs to the recipient. The other anastomotic sites are the ascending aorta, superior and inferior vena cava, and the PA. Mitral annuloplasty ring will be seen posteriorly immediately superior to the base of the mitral leaflet and is rounded in cross-section. Classical maze or radiofrequency maze performed for atrial fibrillation does not generally result in such ridge-like projections. The upper ventricular septum does not have a thin scooped-out appearance to suggest septal resection.

12. **Answer: C.**
Tricuspid valve prolapse. The density of the signal depends on the number of scatterers or the amount of regurgitant flow at the time the signal is generated. The increasing density of the signal from early to late systole suggests an

increasing regurgitant volume through systole, which typically occurs in valve prolapse. In severe pulmonary hypertension, not only will the TR velocity be in the vicinity of 4 m/s but there is no differential signal density. Here, the TR velocity reflects normal PA pressure. The flail valve causes severe TR from the very beginning of systole.

13. **Answer: A.**
PDA. This is the classic appearance of PDA with communication between the distal arch and the origin of the left PA. This view is helpful in diagnosing PDA as well as evaluating the morphology, length, and diameter of the PDA, which are important for planning percutaneous PDA closure.

14. **Answer: D.**
Endomyocardial fibrosis. There is complete obliteration of the left ventricular apex and this associated with hypereosinophilia is suggestive of eosinophilic myocarditis resulting in obliterative thrombofibrotic process in the apex. The accompanying color flow image shows the color stopping short of the apex confirming the obliteration. In apical hypertrophic cardiomyopathy, the LV cavity will be spade shaped. In noncompaction, color gets in between the trabeculae. The LV apical thrombus generally occurs in association with apical aneurysm and could either be protruding or layered. None of these obliterate the LV apex to the extent seen here.

15. **Answer: D.**
Severe pulmonary hypertension with poor RV function. TR velocity is 4 m/s. This is consistent with an RA–RV gradient of 64 mmHg and PA systolic pressure of 80 mmHg in the absence of pulmonary stenosis. A very slow rise of TR velocity indicates a slow rise of RV pressure in early systole, suggestive of RV dysfunction. The TR velocity profile lends itself to calculate RV dp/dt. In this patient, the time taken for the TR velocity to rise from 1 to 3 m/s was 160 ms, corresponding to an RV dp/dt of 200 mmHg/s. RV dp/dt depends upon RV contractile function, PA pressure, and LV contractile function. Normal RV dp/dt with normal PA pressure is 200–250 mmHg/s, but rises to 1000 mmHg/s in the presence of severe pulmonary hypertension associated with good RV contractile function.

16. **Answer: C.**
Severe. This is severe as judged by jet size, vena contracta, and proximal isovelocity surface area (PISA) radius. In addition, the two-dimensional image shows lack of tricuspid leaflet coaptation, leading to wide-open TR. The mechanism is tricuspid annular dilatation and hence is functional, probably secondary to previous pulmonary hypertension due to mitral valve disease resulting in RV and RA dilatation, thus stretching the tricuspid annulus. This is repairable with tricuspid annuloplasty. Also note the partly seen mitral prosthesis. TR quantitations by using the three components of the jet are not well validated.

17. **Answer: C.**
Moderate or severe pulmonary hypertension. In patients with wide-open TR, the tricuspid valve may be fairly nonrestrictive, allowing RV and RA to behave virtually as a single chamber during systole. In such a situation, the TR pressure gradient cannot reliably be calculated using the simplified Bernoulli equation as a considerable amount of energy may be expended in causing acceleration of the TR jet. In addition, RA pressure may be very high, leading to underestimation of PA pressure. In this example, one can count the number of aliases to estimate the

TR velocity at the vena contracta. There are four aliases corresponding to a velocity of 69×4, that is, 2.76 cm/s. Although the pressure gradient is 30 mmHg, the patient is likely to have very high RA pressure, that is, 20–30 mmHg, and because of wide-open TR the TR pressure gradient would have underestimated the pressure gradient. Hence, the PA systolic pressure is at least moderate but more likely to be in the severe range in the absence of pulmonary stenosis. In such patients careful examination of the pulmonary regurgitant jet to get an estimate of PA diastolic pressure would be helpful.

18. **Answer: D.**
Replacement with a mechanical valve. This prosthesis probably is a bileaflet valve in view of the two areas of reverberations seen in the left atrium. A bioprosthetic valve would show struts in the periphery and thin leaflets in the center unless calcified. An annuloplasty ring is an echo dense structure at the base of the mitral leaflet on the left atrial side with intact leaflets. This ring can be partial or complete. An Alfieri stitch can be central or asymmetric and is simply a stitch that focally unites the tips of anterior and posterior leaflets and converts the mitral orifice into a double orifice, best seen in short axis view.

19. **Answer: D.**
All of the above. Preintervention mitral flow is indicative of high left atrial pressure. This pattern is seen despite a heart rate of 92/min, as faster heart rates result in atrial predominance of ventricular filling. Postintervention mitral flow is suggestive of impaired left ventricular relaxation, which is consistent with normal or low mean left atrial pressure. Note that the heart rate is slower at 62/min. This patient had dilated cardiomyopathy with severe functional MR, which responded to diuresis and afterload reduction with a reduction of LV size and elimination of MR. Uncontrolled hypertension will reduce LV ejection performance, increase LV size, and give rise to MR, as myopathic ventricles are exquisitely sensitive to afterload. As these patients have little or no functional reserve, anemia has a serious and deleterious effect on hemodynamics because of a reduction in oxygen-carrying capacity and a demand for higher cardiac output.

20. **Answer: A.**
Thoracic aortic aneurysm. Thoracic aorta runs posterior to the left atrium, is rounded, and on dynamic imaging is pulsatile. Turning the imaging plane by 90 degrees would show the long axis of the descending aorta. The membrane of Cor triatriatum separates the pulmonary venous chamber from the lower part of the atrium and is best seen from parasternal long axis and apical views. The location is across the left atrium. Left PA is not seen in the posterior mediastinum.

20

Questions

1. The commonest location of this pathology is:

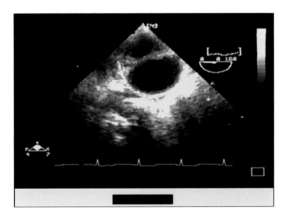

    A. Proximal ascending aorta
    B. Mid-aortic arch
    C. At the attachment of ligamentum arteriosum
    D. Junction of thoracic and abdominal aorta

2. This is a 27-year-old man with no prior medical history, presented with a three-month history of abdominal distension and lower extremity edema. Physical examination revealed severely elevated jugular venous pressure. He had normal left ventricular (LV) and right ventricular (RV) systolic functions. The most likely diagnosis is:

Echocardiography Board Review: 600 Multiple Choice Questions with Discussion, Third Edition.
Ramdas G. Pai and Padmini Varadarajan.
© 2025 John Wiley & Sons Ltd. Published 2025 by John Wiley & Sons Ltd.

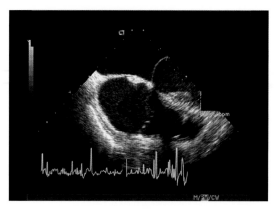

A. Superior mediastinum syndrome
B. Constrictive pericarditis
C. Restrictive cardiomyopathy
D. Cirrhosis of the liver

3. This patient presented with shortness of breath and cyanosis. The most likely cause is:

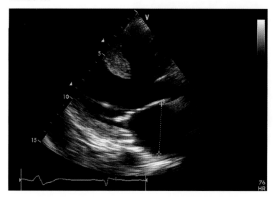

A. Ventricular septal defect (VSD) with Eisenmenger's
B. Atrial septal defect with Eisenmenger's
C. Tetralogy of Fallot
D. Primary pulmonary hypertension

4. This pulmonary regurgitation (PR) signal is suggestive of:

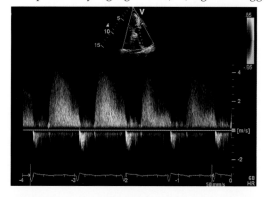

A. Severe pulmonary hypertension
B. Mild pulmonary hypertension
C. Normal pulmonary artery (PA) pressure
D. Severe pulmonic stenosis

5. The Doppler signals shown here are indicative of:

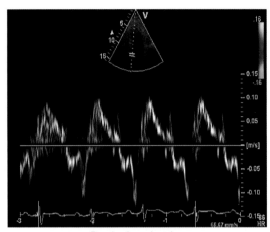

Doppler tissue imaging

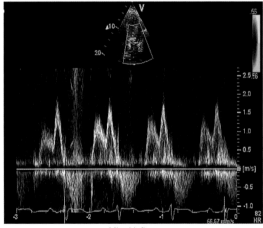

Mitral inflow

A. Normal LV diastolic function
B. Abnormal LV relaxation with probable elevated left atrial (LA) pressure
C. Abnormal LV relaxation with probably normal LA pressure
D. Advanced restrictive cardiomyopathy

6. The continuous wave Doppler signal shown here is suggestive of:

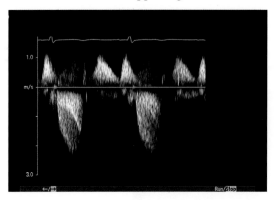

A. Dynamic left ventricular outflow tract (LVOT) obstruction due to systolic anterior motion (SAM)

B. Critical valvular aortic stenosis (AS)

C. Subvalvular AS due to a membrane

D. Flow in and out of pseudoaneurysm

7. This signal was obtained from a right upper parasternal location with the patient turned to the right using a dedicated continuous wave Pedoff transducer. The likely diagnosis is:

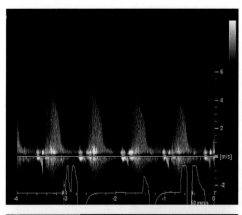

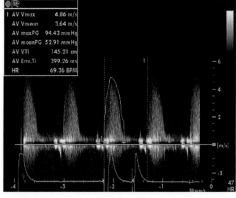

A. Severe mitral regurgitation (MR)
B. Severe tricuspid regurgitation (TR)
C. Severe AS
D. None of the above

8. The aortic valve shown in this image is:

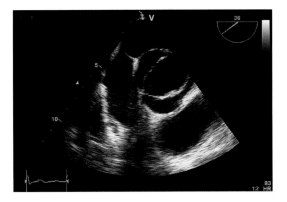

A. Unicuspid
B. Tricuspid
C. Bicuspid
D. Quadricuspid

9. A 32-year-old female with complaints of shortness of breath, pedal edema, flushing, and diarrhea had an echocardiogram. The representative end systolic and end diastolic frame of an RV inflow view is shown. What does the patient have?

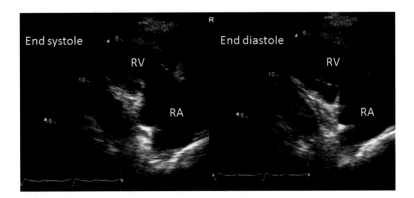

A. Tricuspid valve prolapse potentially causing severe TR
B. Rheumatic involvement of the tricuspid valve
C. Carcinoid involvement of the tricuspid valve
D. None of the above

10. This flow obtained from the distal aortic arch from the suprasternal notch is indicative of:

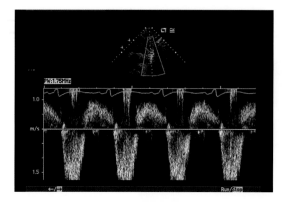

    A. Severe aortic regurgitation (AR)
    B. Aortic coarctation
    C. Severe AS
    D. None of the above

11. This image of the LV is indicative of:

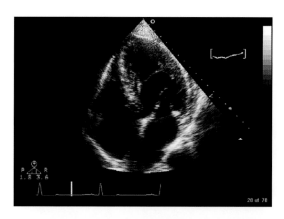

    A. An LA thrombus
    B. LV noncompaction
    C. Bilobed LV
    D. False tendon

12. Saline contrast echocardiography is suggestive of:

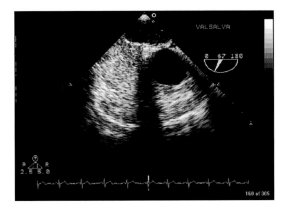

    A. Patent foramen ovale (PFO)
    B. Pulmonary AV fistula
    C. Patent foramen or pulmonary AV fistula
    D. No right to left shunting

13. This transesophageal echocardiogram (TEE) image from the upper esophageal location shows:

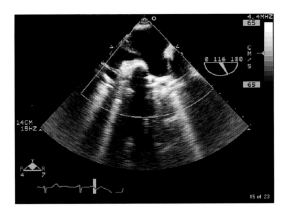

    A. LA appendage
    B. Left upper and lower pulmonary veins
    C. LA and right atrium (RA)
    D. Pulmonary artery branches

14. These two images obtained from the suprasternal notch are diagnostic of:

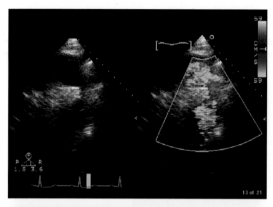

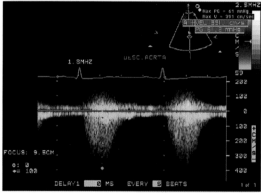

A. Coarctation of the aorta
B. Patent ductus arteriosus
C. Normal aortic flow
D. Pulmonary artery branch stenosis

15. This TEE image is indicative of:

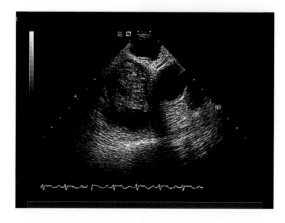

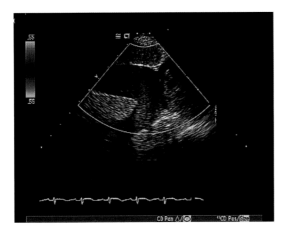

- A. LA myxoma
- B. RA myxoma
- C. Lipomatous atrial septum
- D. Vegetation of the tricuspid valve

16. What is the abnormality seen on this transthoracic echocardiogram?

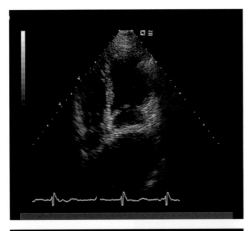

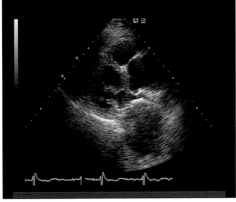

A. Aneurysmal LA
B. Partial absence of the pericardium
C. Thoracic aortic aneurysm
D. Loculated pleural effusion

17. The amount of MR in this patient is likely to be:

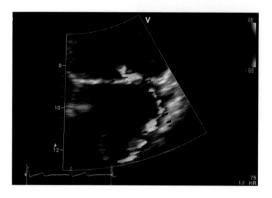

A. 1+
B. 2+
C. 3 or 4+
D. Cannot quantify

18. The cause of the systolic murmur in this patient is likely to be:

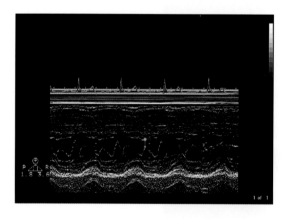

A. Rheumatic MR
B. Valvular AS
C. Hypertrophic obstructive cardiomyopathy (HOCM)
D. Aortic subvalvular membrane

19. This flow was obtained from the LV outflow tract from the apical view using pulse wave Doppler. This patient is most likely to have:

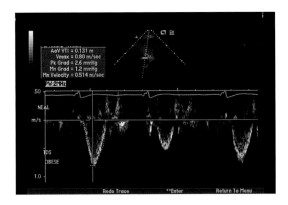

- A. Severe congestive heart failure
- B. Cardiac tamponade
- C. Constrictive pericarditis
- D. HOCM

20. This TEE image is indicative of:

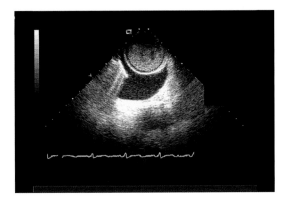

- A. LA thrombus
- B. Aortic dissection
- C. Saccular aneurysm of the aorta with a thrombus
- D. Aortic pseudoaneurysm

Answers for Chapter 20

1. **Answer: C.**
   At the attachment of the ligamentum arteriosum. This is a classic appearance of aortic transection with partial circumference disruption of the aortic wall. In a complete transection there will be discontinuity of the aortic lumen and absence of lower limb pulses. Transection generally is fatal with immediate exsanguination into the mediastinum and the range of presentation includes discovery on TEE after a deceleration injury at one extreme to immediate death at the other extreme. The commonest location is at the junction of the arch and descending aorta where the ligamentum arteriosum is attached. Rarely, it occurs at the arch ascending aortic junction because of differential mobility of these three segments of the aorta and their attachments during rapid deceleration, as in a motor vehicle accident. In aortic dissection the intimal flap is thinner and the rounded shape of the aortic lumen is generally maintained. A mirror image artifact is on the far side of the aorta.

2. **Answer: B.**
   Constrictive pericarditis. This image shows marked pericardial thickening around the RA. On dynamic imaging, the RA wall was tethered to the pericardium along with classic signs of constriction, including septal bounce, respirophasic variations on transvalvular flows, preserved myocardial Em velocity, and global pericardial thickening. His symptoms and physical signs resolved completely after pericardial stripping.

3. **Answer: A.**
   VSD with Eisenmenger's. There is a large VSD. Because of the size, this is nonrestrictive and resulted in a large left to right shunt resulting in pulmonary hypertension. There is no overriding aorta here to suggest tetralogy of Fallot.

4. **Answer: A.**
   Severe pulmonary hypertension. The PR pressure profile reflects a PA to RV diastolic pressure gradient. Hence this patient's PA end systolic pressure is the square of early diastolic PR velocity + RV diastolic pressure, which would be similar to the RA pressure. In this patient this is calculated to be in the range of 80 mmHg, which would also be similar to the mean PA pressure. The PR end diastolic velocity is about 3 m/s. Hence the PA diastolic pressure is 36 + RA pressure. This patient does not have significant pulmonary stenosis, as is shown by the accompanying systolic flow. In fact, a markedly reduced duration is indicative of low cardiac output as well as a consequence of pulmonary hypertension.

5. **Answer: B.**
   An E' of < 8 cm/s and an E/A ratio of < 1 are indicative of abnormal LV relaxation. In addition, the mitral E/annular Em velocity ratio is 24. Normally this is in the range of 8–12. A ratio of > 15 is generally indicative of high LA pressure. However, this is applicable only in the absence of mitral stenosis. E-wave deceleration in this patient does not suggest mitral stenosis. The velocities were increased due to high cardiac output secondary to anemia. Advanced restrictive cardiomyopathy results in a much higher E/A ratio and a rapid E-wave deceleration (< 150 ms).

6. **Answer: A.**
   This late peaking ejection signal, which classically occurs due to dynamic LVOT obstruction due to SAM, occurs in HOCM. SAM is not specific for HOCM as it can occur in situations like postmitral valve repair, volume contracted states,

hyperdynamic LV, and severe mitral annulus calcification. Also note a lower velocity late peaking systolic signal inside the main signal. This is indicative of cavity obliteration and hence a hyperdynamic LV. Valvular AS and fixed subvalvular AS can result in a late peaking signal when they are severe or critical. A relatively low velocity signal in the presence of hyperdynamic LV and mitral flow suggestive of good LV filling are against this possibility.

7. **Answer: C.**
Severe AS. This is a classic signal resulting from severe AS with the flow directed toward the transducer. The timing of the signal is during ejection, as opposed to MR and TR signals that start earlier during systole, and also is less likely to pick up MR and TR signals from this location. This signal shown here is late peaking with a mean gradient of 53 mmHg indicative of severe or critical AS.

8. **Answer: C.**
Bicuspid. This TEE image shows a bicuspid valve with anterior and posterior cusps. The anterior cusp is a conjoint one of right and left cusps. Two commissures can be seen and these should be traced to the annulus to count the number of cusps, as many bicuspid valves have partial commissural fusion only toward the annulus. In fact, it has been shown in a pathology series that nearly 50% of so-called calcific AS cases are bicuspid. These patients may also have ascending aortic dilatation and there is association with coarctation of the aorta. Bicuspid aortic valve is common and occurs in 1–2% of the general population and needs endocarditis prophylaxis. Careful short axis evaluation of the aortic valve is mandatory for every patient referred for echocardiography.

9. **Answer: C.**
The endsystolic and end diastolic frames of the heart show a thickened and retracted tricuspid valve with severely limited mobility suggesting fibrotic process. This is suggestive of carcinoid syndrome, especially in the light of clinical features of diarrhea and flushing. Rheumatic process and fen-phen valvulopathy may look similar, but diarrhea and flushing are not features of these. There is tricuspid valve prolapse in the systolic frame.

10. **Answer: A.**
Severe AR. There is a prominent holodiastolic flow reversal indicative of a retrograde flow in the aorta, indicating diastolic runoff of blood from the arch or the ascending aorta. The conditions that can cause this include significant AR, aorto-pulmonary window, ruptured sinus of Valsalva, fistulous communication to any of the cardiac chambers from the aorta, and large coronary A–V fistula. Coarctation of the aorta may result in diastolic antegrade flow because of collaterals.

11. **Answer: D.**
This is a typical appearance of a false tendon running in the middle of the LV with no pathological significance. When such tendons are present in the apex they can be mistaken for thrombi, and when these run along the anterior septum the thickness of the septum can be overestimated erroneously. This patient does not have significant LV trabeculation either in depth or extent to qualify for noncompaction. Although not all LV segments are shown, significant trabeculation denotes a noncompacted to compacted wall thickness ratio of 2.

12. **Answer: C.**

    There are bubbles in the LA indicative of a right to left shunt. However, from a single frame the level of shunting cannot be determined. Hence the timing of appearance of bubbles in the LA in relation to their appearance in the RA is important. It is important to record at least 8–10 beats after the appearance of contrast in the RA. If the bubbles in the LA appear within 2–3 beats of their appearance in the RA, the shunt probably is at the atrial level; if they appear later, it is likely to be transpulmonary shunting due to pulmonary A–V fistulae. Examples of the latter include end-stage liver disease and Rendu–Weber–Osler disease. In our laboratory we perform saline contrast echo without and with Valsalva's maneuver. The shunt in PFO is conditional to the transient rise in the RA pressure and is produced by Valsalva, coughing, and pressure over the abdomen. Movement of the atrial septum to the left ascertains a higher RA pressure. The PFO diagnosis rate is higher by TEE and with lower limb contrast injection, as the direction of the PFO channel is directly in line with the inferior vena cava (IVC). Hence, injection from the upper limb may be washed away by IVC flow and prevented from entering the PFO channel.

13. **Answer: B.**

    Left upper and lower pulmonary veins. A tomographic plane around 100–120 degrees with the imaging plane superior and left of the appendage shows both left-sided pulmonary veins draining into the LA. Part of the image to the imager's right is cephalad and hence this is the left upper and the one on the right is the left lower pulmonary vein. The ability to get this image depends upon atrial size, pulmonary vein locations, relation of the pulmonary veins to the esophagus, body habitus, etc., but it should be obtainable in over 90% of the patients. The LA appendage is a blind pouch.

14. **Answer: A.**

    Coarctation of the aorta. This is a classic image of coarctation of the aorta. The two-dimensional image shows narrowing at the junction of the arch and descending aorta with turbulence on color flow imaging. The flow velocity across this narrowing was 3.9 m/s, indicative of a systolic gradient of 61 mmHg. This is indicative of severe coarctation. Other indicators of severity include a broader systolic signal, diastolic gradient, and nonpulsatile flow in the descending aorta. Presence of arterial collaterals may reduce the gradient but the collateral-dependent flow in the descending aorta will be nonpulsatile.

15. **Answer: B.**

    Right atrial myxoma. In this image there is clearly a right atrial mass, which is very large. Also note a very dilated IVC with no mass inside. The differential diagnosis includes myxoma, thrombus, and metastatic tumor spreading through the IVC, such as renal cell carcinoma. The features that help to differentiate it are attachment of the mass (pedunculated attachment to the septum, likely to be myxoma), continuity of the mass in the IVC (renal cell carcinoma), presence of blood vessels in the mass on color flow (not a thrombus), and presence of perfusion by transpulmonary contrast agents (thrombus has no enhancement, myxoma has mild enhancement, vascular tumors hyperenhance). This mass is too big for valve vegetation.

16. **Answer: C.**

    Thoracic aortic aneurysm. The structure behind the LA is the thoracic aorta, which is normally seen in the parasternal long axis view. The long axis of this part of the aorta can be visualized from the left parasternal view with the left parasagittal imaging plane.

17. **Answer: C.**
3 or 4+. This patient has a lateral wall-hugging jet reaching all the way to the roof of the LA. A wall-hugging jet area tends to be 40–50% smaller than a free jet area for a given regurgitant volume. In such patients, examining the size of the vena contracta, the proximal isovelocity surface area (PISA), and calculating the effective regurgitant orifice area would be helpful for volumetric quantitation. Although the PISA is not well visualized in this patient, the diameter of the vena contracta is about 5 mm, which is consistent with at least 3+ mitral regurgitation. The mechanism of the lateral wall-hugging jet in this patient was a tethered posterior leaflet secondary to a rheumatic process. The other mechanism to cause a laterally directed jet would be a severely prolapsing anterior mitral leaflet.

18. **Answer: C.**
HOCM. This is a typical M mode of systolic anterior motion of the mitral valve. The CD segment of the mitral valve (systolic segment) normally moves anteriorly during systole because of the translation of the LV and mitral valve anteriorly. However, a CD segment slope greater than the slope of the posterior endocardium and the systolic mitral leaflet septal contact indicates SAM, which most commonly occurs in HOCM but can occur in other situations too. The mitral valve opening is normal in this patient with a normal ejection fraction slope with thin leaflets ruling out rheumatic mitral stenosis. Fixed aortic stenosis due to a valvular or subvalvular process does not give rise to any typical appearance of the mitral valve.

19. **Answer: A.**
Severe congestive heart failure. The beat in the middle is of lesser amplitude and duration, which gives a markedly lower time velocity integral compared to the beats on either side. Note that the R–R intervals are regular. A lower stroke volume and a weaker pulse with every other beat is called pulsus alternans and is suggestive of severe left ventricular systolic dysfunction. The change in amplitude is too rapid for respirophasic variation, which occurs in tamponade and constriction. Pulsus alternans is not seen in HOCM as it is mostly diastolic dysfunction and the LVOT velocity is higher because of SAM-related flow acceleration.

20. **Answer: B.**
Aortic dissection. This is a transverse section through the descending thoracic aorta. A smaller true lumen and a larger false lumen with a thrombus are seen. Also note the fluid around the aorta that is indicative of left pleural effusion and this should raise the possibility of a leaking aneurysm. During dissection or intramural hematoma, the thrombus is inside the aortic wall and is covered by the endothelium, as in this case. In a saccular aneurysm with an intraluminal thrombus, the endothelium is outside the thrombus. Pseudoaneurysm is characterized by an aneurysm bound only by adventitia outside the aortic lumen and communicating with the aorta through a narrow neck.

21

Questions

1. This patient is likely to have:

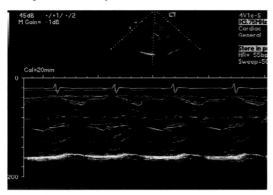

A. Mitral valve prolapse
B. Elevated left ventricular end diastolic pressure (LVEDP)
C. Hypertrophic obstructive cardiomyopathy (HOCM)
D. Severe aortic regurgitation (AR)

2. The mitral valve motion in this patient suggests:

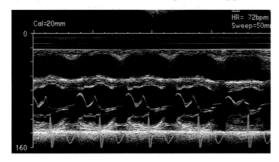

Echocardiography Board Review: 600 Multiple Choice Questions with Discussion, Third Edition.
Ramdas G. Pai and Padmini Varadarajan.
© 2025 John Wiley & Sons Ltd. Published 2025 by John Wiley & Sons Ltd.

A. Atrial fibrillation
B. Elevated LVEDP
C. Mitral valve prolapse
D. Severe AR

3. The aortic valve M mode is suggestive of:

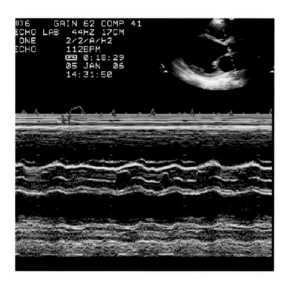

A. Aortic stenosis
B. HOCM
C. Congestive heart failure
D. Hypertension

4. Flow in the abdominal aorta in this patient is indicative of:

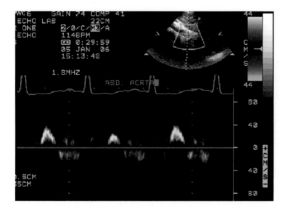

A. Systolic heart failure
B. Severe coarctation of aorta
C. Severe AR
D. Large patent ductus arteriosus (PDA)

5. The continuous wave Doppler signal is suggestive of:

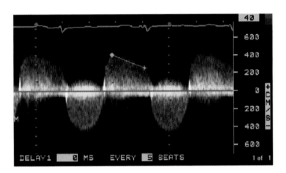

A. Severe mixed aortic valve disease
B. Mixed pulmonary valve disease
C. Mixed mitral valve disease
D. Mitral and AR

6. This patient is likely to have:

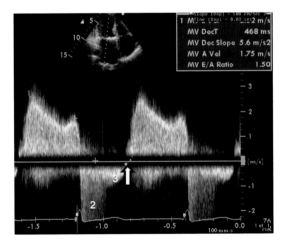

A. Mild AR
B. Mitral stenosis (MS) with high left atrial (LA) pressure
C. Acute severe AR
D. Severe mitral regurgitation (MR)

7. This patient has mitral stenosis with:

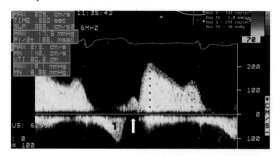

   A. High LA pressure
   B. Hyperdynamic left ventricle (LV)
   C. Severe LV systolic dysfunction
   D. MR

8. The continuous wave Doppler signal is suggestive of:

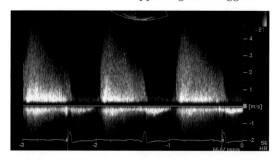

   A. Mild MS
   B. Severe MS
   C. Mild AR
   D. Severe AR

9. The continuous wave Doppler signal is suggestive of:

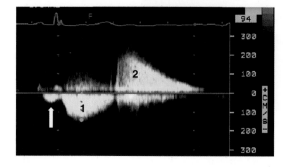

   A. Severe AR
   B. MS
   C. Pulmonary hypertension
   D. Severe pulmonary regurgitation (PR)

10. This patient has:

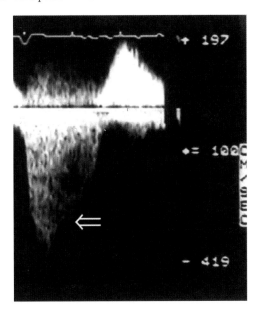

A. Mild to moderate aortic stenosis
B. Mild MR
C. Acute severe MR
D. Ventral septal defect (VSD) with pulmonary hypertension

11. The cause of systolic murmur in this patient is likely to be:

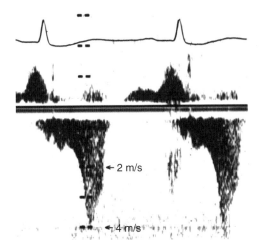

A. HOCM
B. Valvular aortic stenosis
C. Mitral valve prolapse
D. VSD

12. This continuous wave signal in a 22-year-old woman with a history of heart surgery during infancy is indicative of:

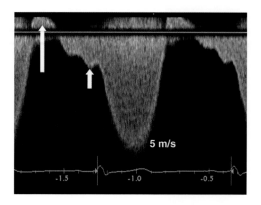

5 m/s

A. Severe aortic stenosis
B. Severe pulmonary stenosis (PS)
C. Severe PS and regurgitation
D. Severe pulmonary hypertension

13. This patient has:

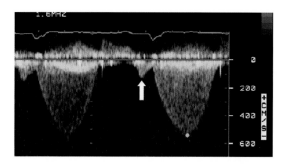

A. Severe PS
B. Normal pulmonary artery (PA) pressure
C. Both of the above
D. Neither of the above

14. The signal indicated by the arrow is produced by:

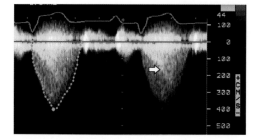

A. Valvular PS
B. Dynamic subvalvular PS on top of valvular PS
C. MR
D. VSD

15. This signal was obtained from:

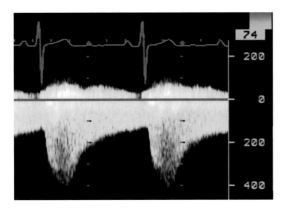

A. Apical window
B. Parasternal window
C. Suprasternal window
D. Subcostal window

16. This patient has:

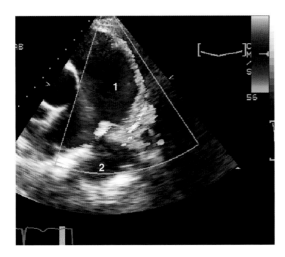

A. PA branch stenosis
B. PR
C. PDA
D. None of the above

17. This continuous wave signal is indicative of:

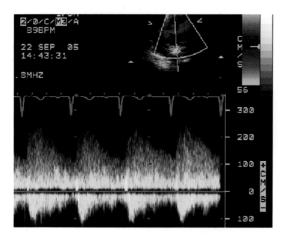

   A. Severe AR
   B. PDA
   C. Coarctation of the aorta
   D. Atrial septal defect (ASD) flow

18. The flow obtained on transesophageal echocardiogram (TEE) from a descending thoracic aorta is indicative of:

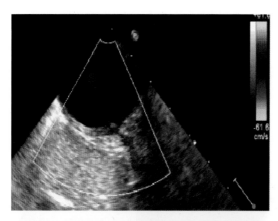

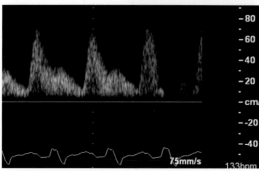

A. Aortic coarctation
B. PDA
C. Normal flow in intercostal artery
D. Severe AR

19. Flow from this subcostal view is indicative of:

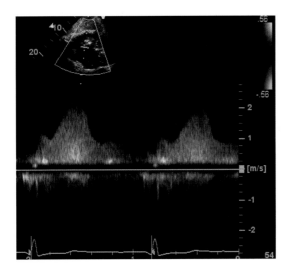

A. Large ASD
B. Severe MR
C. MS
D. Tricuspid stenosis

20. This was a recording of flow across the pulmonary valve using pulsed wave Doppler in a patient with severe dyspnea. The likely diagnosis is:

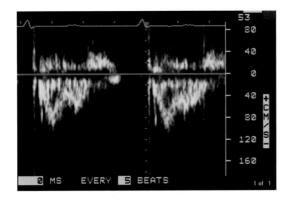

A. Pulmonary hypertension
B. PS
C. PR
D. Large ASD

Answers for Chapter 21

1. **Answer: C.**
   HOCM. Note the systolic anterior motion (SAM) of the anterior mitral leaflet starting in mid systole. SAM narrows the LV outflow tract in a dynamic manner producing LV outflow obstruction and gradient. Elevated LVEDP is not an unreasonable response as deceleration of mitral A-wave is slow, although not a classic B hump. Mitral valve prolapse results in late systolic sagging of mitral valve not anterior motion. Severe AR with a posteriorly directed jet onto the anterior mitral leaflet results in diastolic fluttering.

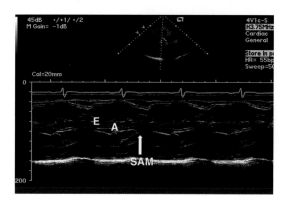

2. **Answer: B.**
   Elevated LVEDP. Note the prominent B hump after the A point of mitral valve motion. In atrial fibrillation there is loss of A-wave. Also see the explanation for Question 1.

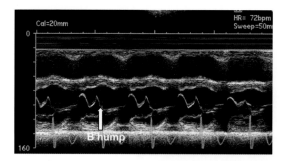

3. **Answer: C.**
   Congestive heart failure. This is typical of pulsus alternans, which occurs in severe systolic heart failure. Note that there is reduced opening and duration of opening of the aortic valve with every other beat, and this results from reduced stroke volume with every other beat. Also note that in this instance, pulsus alternans was triggered by a premature ventricular complex. In aortic stenosis there is leaflet

thickening and reduced opening. In HOCM there may be mid-systolic closure of the aortic valve. Hypertension does not produce any characteristic changes in aortic valve motion.

4. **Answer: A.**
Systolic heart failure. This is consistent with pulsus alternans. See the explanation for Question 403. In severe aortic coarctation, collateral-dependent flow will produce continuous flow without pulsatility. In severe AR and large PDA, runoff of flow from aorta into LV and PA, respectively, during diastole produces diastolic retrograde flow.

5. **Answer: A.**
Severe mixed aortic valve disease. The systolic signal starts several milliseconds after the onset of QRS complex, suggestive of origin at the aortic or pulmonary valve, that is, flow during the ejection phase. Flow at atrioventricular valves due to regurgitation starts earlier during the isovolumic contraction period and extends into the isovolumic relaxation period too. Hence it will overlap the AR signal, which occupies both these isovolumic phases as well. The systolic and diastolic signals are continuous with each other, suggesting origin at the same valve. A mid-peaking systolic signal of > 4 m/s is suggestive of severe aortic stenosis. High diastolic velocity is also not compatible with MS. Severe PS is generally incompatible with severe pulmonary hypertension – hence severe PS and PR are not possible as a high velocity PR signal occurs only with severe pulmonary hypertension.

6. **Answer: B.**
MS with high LA pressure. The diastolic signal (1) is that of MS and this patient is in sinus rhythm as there is an A-wave. The peak diastolic gradient is about 30 mmHg and the mean gradient is 18 mmHg at a heart rate of 76 beats/min, which is indicative of severe MS. The arrow points to isovolumic relaxation time (IVRT), which was 30 ms indicating high LA pressure or large left atrial "V"-wave. Signal (2) indicates partial MR velocity as it is contiguous with the ending of the MS signal and (3) indicates LV outflow and the gap between that and mitral inflow, which is indicated by the arrow in IVRT.

7. **Answer: B.**
Hyperdynamic LV. The systolic signal denoted by "1" is not MR but is due to LV cavity obliteration as it is late peaking and hence indicates a hyperdynamic LV. It also occurs during ejection phase, unlike the MR signal. IVRT indicated by the arrow is 110 ms (time between small marks is 200 ms and between two vertical lines is 1 s) and this indicates normal LA pressure. IVRT is the Doppler equivalent of the auscultatory A2–OS interval, that is, the interval between the aortic component of the second heart sound and the opening snap in MS. A short A2–OS interval indicates severe MS.

8. **Answer: D.**
Severe AR. The velocity is too high for MS as such a high transmitral gradient is not compatible with life. Rapid deceleration of AR signal indicates rapidly diminishing aortic to LV diastolic gradient as diastole progresses. This may occur either due to rapidly dropping aortic pressure or increasing LV diastolic pressure. These occur in severe or acute severe AR, respectively. In severe MS the signal decelerates slowly.

9. **Answer: D.**

Severe PR. Signal no. 2 is early diastolic following ejection flow no. 1 suggestive of origin at a semilunar valve. The arrow points to forward flow across the semilunar valve with atrial systole and this can occur only at the pulmonary valve with normal PA pressure. If the PA pressure is high, atrial systole cannot generate a forward flow even when there is late diastolic equilibration of pressures between PA, RV, and RA. For the same reason, you do not get forward flow across the aortic valve in severe AR as aortic diastolic pressure is too high, and high LV diastolic pressure may cause premature closure of the mitral valve. The diastolic flow is of low velocity and ends in mid diastole, indicating severe PR with normal PA pressure.

10. **Answer: C.**

Acute severe MR. This is a classic "V"-wave cutoff sign of MR with rapid deceleration of the MR signal due to a large left atrial "V"-wave resulting in a rapid reduction in the pressure gradient between LV and LA in late systole. This occurs typically in acute severe MR, as in papillary muscle rupture or flail mitral valve. It is not an AS signal as it starts with QRS and continues into mitral inflow, indicating an origin at the mitral valve. VSD flow does not have diastolic flow in the opposite direction.

11. **Answer: A.**

HOCM. This is a typical dagger-shaped continuous wave signal that typically occurs in HOCM. That is because of the fact that the obstruction in HOCM is dynamic due to the SAM of the mitral valve and the obstruction is maximum in late systole at the height of SAM–septal contact. This results in the highest gradient in late systole. In mitral valve prolapse, although MR is more in late systole, the LV–LA pressure gradient is highest in mid systole. In severe valvular AS the signal could be late peaking, but there would be a gap between mitral flow and valvular AS signal (the gap due to the LV isovolumic contraction period). In intraventricular obstructions as in HOCM, the signal of dynamic LVOT obstruction is continuous with mitral inflow.

12. **Answer: C.**

Severe PS and regurgitation. This patient in fact had a bovine jugular nonvalved conduit between RV and PA for pulmonary atresia in a foreign country during infancy and presented with shortness of breath and edema. As the conduit has become too small for her body size and flow requirements, it was functionally stenotic resulting in a very high systolic gradient. The longer arrow points to the PR signal. The PR is severe and also it rapidly decelerates with equilibration of pressures between PA and RV. The shorter arrow indicates forward flow with right atrial systole, which indicates normal PA pressure.

13. **Answer: C.**

Both are true. This patient has severe PS: the peak systolic gradient is closer to 90 mmHg. It is not an AS or MR signal as there is forward flow with atrial systole (arrow) and this also indicates normal PA pressure. Low PR velocity, seen here, also confirms normal PA diastolic pressure.

14. **Answer: B.**

Dynamic subvalvular PS on top of valvular PS. The late peaking signal was due to muscular dynamic subvalvular PS on top of valvular PS shown by the signal, which is being measured on the first beat. In such a patient one has to volume-load and pretreat the patient with a beta-blocker before balloon valvuloplasty of the pulmonary valve to prevent a "suicide right ventricle." The latter may occur due to an excessively hyperdynamic RV following relief of RV afterload by balloon valvuloplasty.

15. **Answer: C.**
    Suprasternal window. This is a classic flow because of severe coarctation of the aorta with systolic and diastolic components. The signals are negative or flow is going away from the transducer. This signal is obtained from the suprasternal window.

16. **Answer: C.**
    PDA. This is a typical PDA flow obtained from a parasternal short axis basal view with clockwise rotation of the probe to show PA and branches. No. 1 indicates the dilated main PA and no. 2 the arch/descending aortic junction from which flow is occurring into the PA. Note that this is a diastolic frame (see marker on ECG) and flow is into the main PA, hence it is not left PA branch stenosis.

17. **Answer: B.**
    PDA. This is a typical PDA flow from a parasternal view with flow from aorta to PA. It is continuous. Note this is a transthoracic image and it is difficult to obtain coarctation flow from below on a transthoracic echocardiogram to yield a positive signal. This may be possible on a TEE. The AR signal will be diastolic only.

18. **Answer: A.**
    Aortic coactation. Note that the flow is into the aortic lumen throughout the cardiac cycle, indicative of retrograde flow in the intercostal artery. This occurs in collateral-dependent distal perfusion as it occurs in severe aortic coarctation. This patient had interrupted aorta. In severe AR, holodiastolic retrograde flow occurs in the aortic lumen.

19. **Answer: B.**
    Severe MR. This flow is across the foramen ovale due to excessive stretching produced by high atrial pressures. The flow is from LA to RA and note that the highest velocity is in late systole, indicative of a large left atrial "V"-wave, which occurs in severe MR. In large ASD flow will be nonrestrictive across the defect, resulting in very low or transient pressure gradients.

20. **Answer: A.**
    Pulmonary hypertension. This is a typical "flying W sign" associated with pulmonary hypertension. Mid-systolic deceleration occurs because of rapidly returning reflected pressure waves secondary to a stiffer PA that occurs when it operates under high pressure. There is no PR signal and no continuous wave signal to assess if there is a gradient across the pulmonary valve. The velocity of the signal is under 1 m/s, indicating a normal amount of pulmonary artery flow, and this is inconsistent with a large ASD. A large ASD is associated with increased pulmonary artery flow.

22

Questions

1. This transesophageal echocardiogram (TEE) image is diagnostic of:

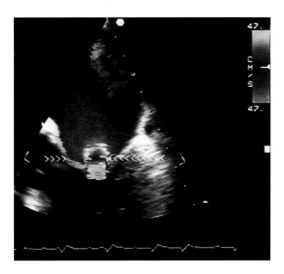

   A. Rheumatic mitral stenosis (MS)
   B. Mitral regurgitation (MR)
   C. Prosthetic valve stenosis
   D. Calcific MS

Echocardiography Board Review: 600 Multiple Choice Questions with Discussion, Third Edition.
Ramdas G. Pai and Padmini Varadarajan.
© 2025 John Wiley & Sons Ltd. Published 2025 by John Wiley & Sons Ltd.

2. LA, left atrium. This transthoracic image is suggestive of:

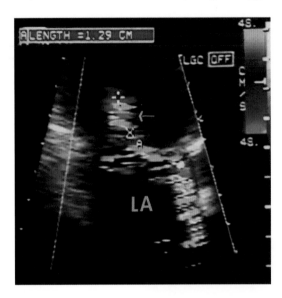

   A. MS
   B. Mild MR
   C. Severe MR due to flail posterior mitral leaflet
   D. Severe MR due to dilated mitral annulus

3. The pulmonary vein flow shown here is suggestive of:

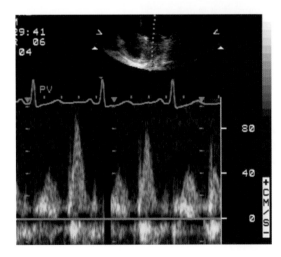

   A. Severe MR
   B. Severe MS
   C. Normal left atrial (LA) pressure
   D. High LA pressure

4. The mitral flow profile and mitral annular velocity in this patient are consistent with:

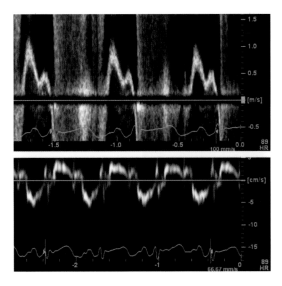

   A. Symptomatic severe MR due to flail mitral valve in a 24-year-old with normal left ventricle (LV) size and function
   B. Class III symptoms in a patient with dilated LV and ejection fraction (EF) of 30%
   C. Normal LV function with mild MR and class I symptoms
   D. Acute severe aortic regurgitation (AR) with left ventricular end diastolic pressure (LVEDP) of 55 mmHg

5. The parasternal short axis view shown here is consistent with:

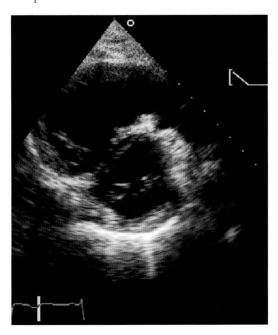

A. Pulmonary hypertension
B. Flail mitral valve
C. Dilated cardiomyopathy
D. None of the above

6. This patient is likely to have:

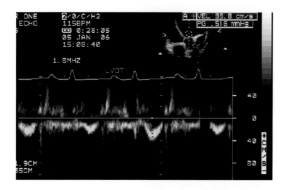

A. Severe LV dysfunction with low cardiac output state
B. AR
C. Hypertrophic obstructive cardiomyopathy (HOCM)
D. None of the above

7. This patient has:

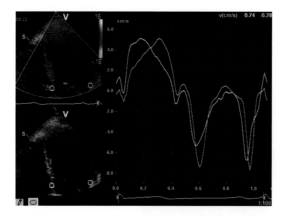

A. LV systolic dyssynchrony
B. LV diastolic dyssynchrony
C. Good LV synchrony
D. None of the above

8. The signals shown here are annular:

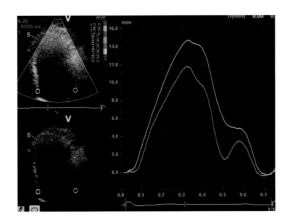

   A. Velocity
   B. Displacement
   C. Strain
   D. Strain rate

9. The signals from septum and LV lateral wall are those of:

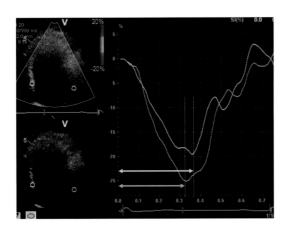

   A. LV strain
   B. Strain rate
   C. Velocity
   D. None of the above

10. The arrows point to:

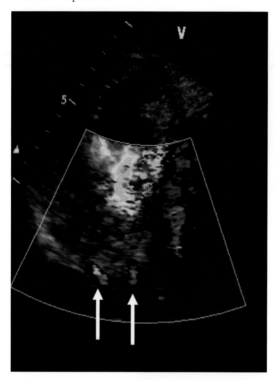

A. Coronary sinus branches
B. Coronary artery branches
C. Artifacts produced by tissue motion
D. None of the above

11. RVOT/LVOT, right/left ventricular outflow tract. Data shown here permit computation of:

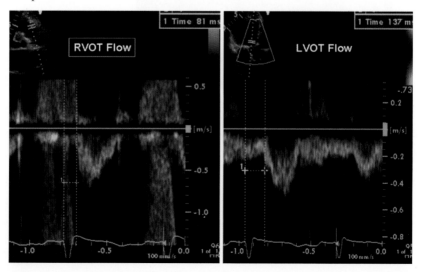

A. LV intraventricular dyssynchrony
B. Interventricular dyssynchrony
C. Atrioventricular (AV) dyssynchrony
D. None of the above

12. In this TEE image, the downward pointing arrow refers to:

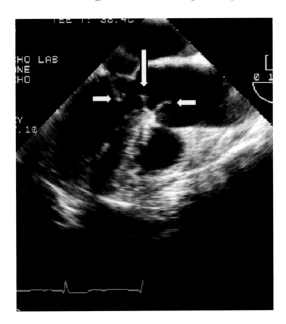

A. Aortic valve
B. Vegetation on the aortic valve
C. Aortic subvalvular membrane
D. Aortic dissection

13. Ao, aorta. The arrow on this TEE image points to:

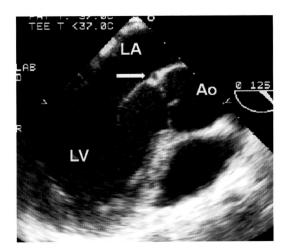

A. Coronary artery
B. Aortic valve ring abscess
C. Artifact
D. Coronary sinus

14. This patient has:

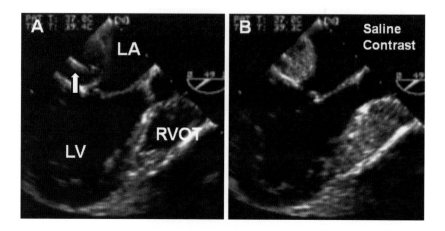

A. Dilated coronary sinus and dextrocardia
B. Dilated coronary sinus and levocardia
C. Cor triatriatum
D. Aneurysm of circumflex coronary artery

15. DTA, descending thoracic aorta. The arrow points to:

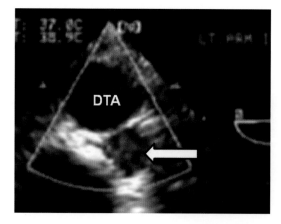

A. Aortic aneurysm
B. Inferior vena cava
C. Dilated azygos vein
D. Mirror image artifact

16. The image shown is indicative of:

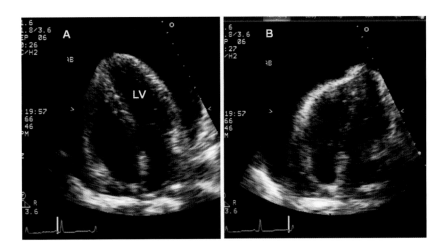

    A. Large left pleural effusion
    B. Cardiac tamponade
    C. Congenital absence of pericardium
    D. Artifact

17. This TEE performed on a patient who presented with acute severe chest pain is indicative of:

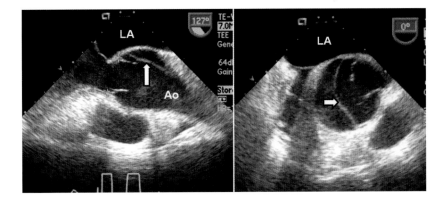

    A. Type A aortic dissection
    B. Type B aortic dissection
    C. A mirror image artifact originating from the right pulmonary artery
    D. Abnormal structure of the aortic valve

18. This TEE image is diagnostic of:

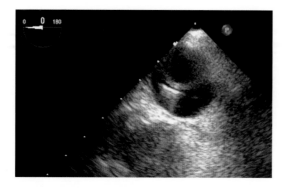

A. Aortic dissection with wire in true lumen
B. Aortic dissection with wire in false lumen
C. Double barrel aorta
D. Aortic stent post endovascular repair

19. This M mode examination is suggestive of:

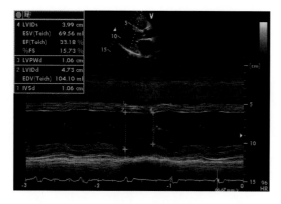

A. Severe LV systolic failure
B. Hypertrophic cardiomyopathy
C. Large pericardial effusion
D. Cardiac amyloidosis

20. The continuous wave Doppler signal from the tricuspid valve is consistent with:

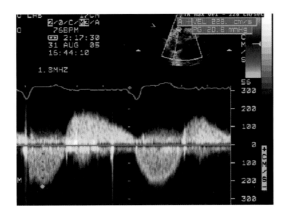

A. Carcinoid syndrome
B. Severe pulmonary hypertension
C. Constriction
D. None of the above

Answers for Chapter 22

1. **Answer: A.**
   Rheumatic MS. The chamber on the top is the LA and note the doming of the anterior mitral leaflet, suggestive of rheumatic MS. Note that the proximal isovelocity surface area (PISA) is on the LA side. This is a native valve without prosthetic valve sewing ring or struts. In degenerative or calcific MS, the annulus is heavily calcified and calcium extends centripetally into the valve leaflets without any commissural fusion. Commissural fusion with pliable leaflets is a prerequisite for doming.

2. **Answer: C.**
   Severe MR due to flail posterior mitral leaflet. The PISA is on the LV side with closed mitral leaflets in systole, suggestive of MR rather than MS. The radius of the PISA is 1.3 cm at a Nyquist limit of 48 cm/s, resulting in a peak instantaneous regurgitant flow rate of $2 \times 3.14 \times (1.3)^2 \times 48$, which equals roughly 500 cc/s, correlating with severe MR (regurgitant flow rate > 200 cc/s = severe MR). MR jet in dilated annulus would be central. A medial wall-hugging jet shown here is consistent with flail posterior mitral leaflet.

3. **Answer: D.**
   High LA pressure. A larger pulmonary vein D-wave with rapid deceleration suggests high LA pressure. A D-wave deceleration time of < 170 ms is indicative of high LA pressure. This could be significant MR, but systolic flow reversal in the pulmonary vein is a definitive sign of severe MR with a large V-wave. In MS the D-wave decelerates slowly, paralleling the E-wave deceleration slope.

4. **Answer: B.**
   Class III symptoms in a patient with dilated LV and EF of 30%. Mitral E/A ratio of 2 and E/Em ratio of 22 are indicative of high LA pressure and likely of class III symptoms. Note that the mitral annular Em velocity is < 5 cm/s and S-wave velocity is 3.5 cm/s, suggestive of both LV diastolic and systolic dysfunction, which are more consistent with an EF of 30% and functional MR (note the MR signal on pulse wave). In acute severe AR with LVEDP of 55 mmHg, there would be premature closure of the mitral valve and absence of mitral A-wave.

5. **Answer: A.**
   Pulmonary hypertension. Note that this is an endsystolic frame (see the ECG marker). The septum is flattened and LV is D-shaped with a large hypertrophied RV. These are indicative of pulmonary hypertension.

6. **Answer: A.**
   Severe LV dysfunction with low cardiac output state. Note that the flow is obtained by placing a pulse wave sample in the LV outflow tract from the apical view. Note that the V1 is < 40 cm/s, suggesting low cardiac output. Although the patient is in sinus rhythm, output with every other beat is less indicative of pulsus alternans, which occurs in severe systolic heart failure.

7. **Answer: A.**
   LV systolic dyssynchrony. Tissue Doppler or tissue velocity images are shown here. Focal velocity profiles of medial (yellow) and lateral annulus (green) are produced offline by placing samples in these regions. Note that the peak of lateral annulus velocity is about 150 ms after the medial annulus velocity peak,

suggestive of septolateral mechanical dyssynchrony. A septolateral delay of > 65 ms is indicative of LV dyssynchrony. There was good diastolic synchrony as judged by annular E-wave velocity profiles.

8. **Answer: B.**

   Displacement. Note that the units are in mm and the signals are toward the apex. Normal mitral annular displacement is 12–17 mm in systole, highest for the lateral annulus and less for the medial annulus. Reduced displacement is indicative of impaired LV long axis function and can occur even in the presence of normal EF and minor axis function.

9. **Answer: A.**

   LV strain. Note that the units are in %, which is % shortening compared to original length. Normal myocardial strain is 15–20%, very similar to % sarcomeric shortening during contraction of cardiac muscle cell.

10. **Answer: A.**

    Coronary sinus branches. These can be obtained from an apical four-chamber view with posterior tilt using preferably power mode on color flow imaging. The blue color indicates flow toward the base and this is indicative of flow in coronary sinus branches. Coronary artery flow would be in the opposite direction.

11. **Answer: B.**

    Interventricular dyssynchrony. The time interval between RV and LV ejection derived from respective flows referenced to the QRS complex is called aortopulmonary mechanical delay and is a measure of interventricular synchrony. The normal is < 40 ms and a value greater than this is indicative of interventricular dyssynchrony. In this example, aortopulmonary mechanical delay is 137 minus 81 or 56 ms. Measures of LV synchrony are obtained from LV myocardial velocity or strain imaging at a high temporal resolution. AV synchrony refers to optimal timing of atrial contraction.

12. **Answer: C.**

    Aortic subvalvular membrane. This is a classic example of membranous subaortic stenosis. Also note part of this circumferential membrane on the LV side of the anterior mitral leaflet. The image also shows the aortic valve (left pointing arrow) and systolic anterior motion of the anterior mitral leaflet (right pointing arrow).

13. **Answer: A.**

    Coronary artery. This was an anomalous circumflex coronary artery originating from the right coronary artery with a retroaortic course between aorta and LA. Note that it is small and perfectly circular, unlike an abscess, which tends to have irregular edges and inflammatory thickening or other sequelae around it. One can study the course of the vessel by imaging this structure in different imaging planes. Coronary sinus would be in the posterior AV groove.

14. **Answer: A.**

    Dilated coronary sinus and dextrocardia. Note opacification of the structure at the AV groove with saline contrast, indicating anomalous connection of left or right or the entire superior vena cava into the coronary sinus (as it is not specified which arm was injected). Also note a pacemaker lead in the coronary sinus. At a 49 degree angle, the left ventricular outflow tract is on the right side, indicating dextrocardia. This view is typically obtained at 120–140 degrees with levocardia – sort of a mirror image.

15. **Answer: C.**
    Dilated azygos vein. This is a typical appearance. This patient had an interrupted inferior vena cava (IVC) and the IVC drained through the azygos vein into the superior vena cava. The IVC does not relate to the thoracic aorta. The mirror image artifact looks like a duplicate image of descending thoracic aorta.

16. **Answer: B.**
    Cardiac tamponade. There is a large pericardial effusion with a swinging heart. Also note electrical alternans in the accompanying ECG. Excessive mobility of the heart is also seen in absent pericardium and this would occur with change in body position and there would not be echo-free space around the heart.

17. **Answer: A.**
    Type A aortic dissection. This is a typical aortic flap and indicative of type A aortic dissection involving ascending aorta. Type B dissection involves descending aorta only.

18. **Answer: B.**
    Aortic dissection with wire in false lumen. This was a patient with acute type A aortic dissection. The true lumen is rounded, the false lumen is outside that, and the wire is in the false lumen. TEE was used to guide antegrade cannulation of the aorta but was unsuccessful because of a very small, compressed true lumen in the ascending aorta. Hence, the aorta had to be cannulated retrogradely.

19. **Answer: A.**
    Severe LV systolic failure. Although the LV is not dilated, there is poor wall thickening and poor reduction in LV size with systole. The LV wall is neither thick nor thick and echoreflective, as you may see in hypertrophic cardiomyopathy or cardiac amyloid, respectively.

20. **Answer: A.**
    Carcinoid syndrome. Note that the patient has both tricuspid regurgitation (TR) and tricuspid stenosis (TS). This combination is consistent with carcinoid involvement of the tricuspid valve. Mixed TR and TS can also be seen with rheumatic heart disease, fen-phen valvulopathy, post-tricuspid repair, or a dysfunctional bioprosthetic tricuspid valve.

23

Questions

1. A 45-year-old female was admitted to the hospital with complaints of acute onset of shortness of breath. This still frame shows:

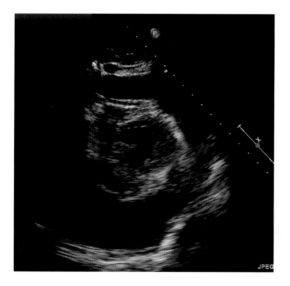

   A. Pleural effusion
   B. Pericardial effusion
   C. Normal heart

Echocardiography Board Review: 600 Multiple Choice Questions with Discussion, Third Edition.
Ramdas G. Pai and Padmini Varadarajan.
© 2025 John Wiley & Sons Ltd. Published 2025 by John Wiley & Sons Ltd.

2. The M mode from the patient in Question 1 shows:

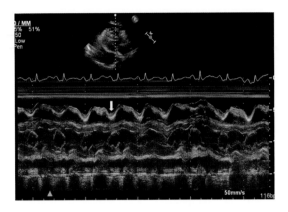

   A. Normal M mode through the heart
   B. Diastolic collapse of the right ventricle
   C. Pericardial thickening

3. The Doppler across the aortic valve shows:

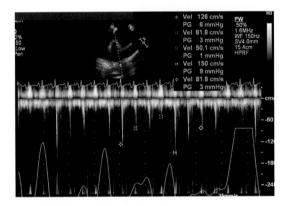

   A. Normal Doppler flow pattern
   B. Tamponade
   C. Restriction

4. The Doppler flow across the pulmonary valve is suggestive of:

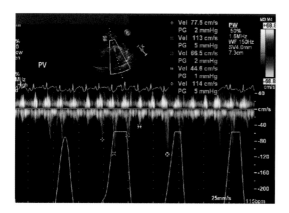

A. Normal flow pattern
B. Restriction
C. Constriction
D. Tamponade

5. The image of the inferior vena cava (IVC) from the patient in Questions 1–4 is suggestive of:

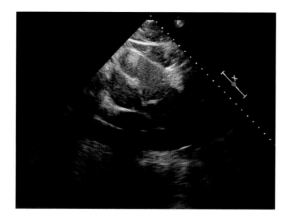

A. Normal right atrial (RA) pressure
B. Low RA pressure
C. Elevated RA pressure

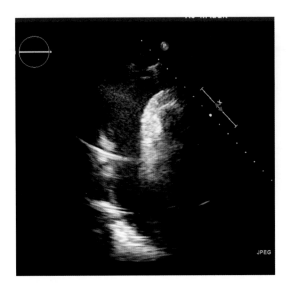

A. Normal appearance of the left ventricle (LV)

B. Catheter in the pleural space

C. Catheter in the pericardial space

7. Two days later, the patient complained of increased shortness of breath. The image shows:

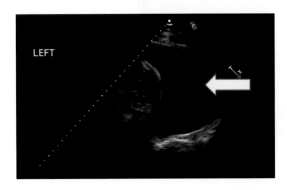

A. Pericardial effusion

B. Pleural effusion

8. The arrow points to:

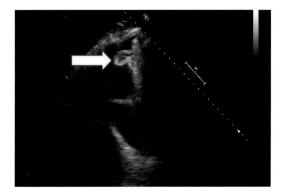

    A. Normal appearance of the myocardium
    B. Masses in the pericardial space
    C. Artifact

9. A 23-year-old female presented with complaints of a sudden onset of severe shortness of breath. She gave a remote history of skin rash. Her labs indicate a eosinophil count of 20%. The most likely diagnosis is:

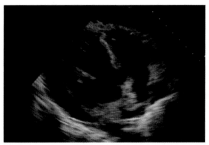 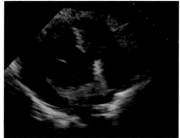

    Diastolic frame   Systolic frame

    A. Constrictive pericarditis
    B. Eosinophilic myocarditis
    C. Giant cell myocarditis

10. A 42-year-old male with a history of Down's syndrome was evaluated with an echocardiogram. The image shows:

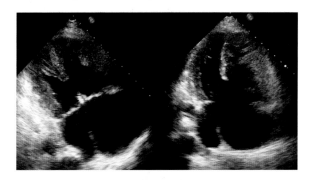

    A. Ventricular septal defect
    B. Atrial septal defect
    C. Partial atrioventricular (AV) canal
    D. Complete AV canal

11. In a 45-year-old male with end-stage liver disease a saline contrast injection was performed. The findings are suggestive of:

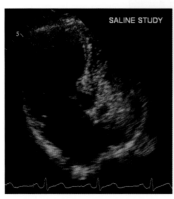 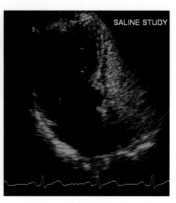

First beat after saline injection   13th beat after saline injection

    A. Right to left shunt across a patent foremen ovale (PFO)
    B. Right to left shunt suggestive of transpulmonary shunt
    C. Left to right shunt
    D. Cannot be determined

12. The arrow shows:

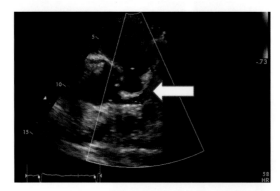

    A. Flow in the pulmonary artery
    B. Flow in the aorta
    C. Coronary blood flow
    D. Cannot determine

13. The arrow points to:

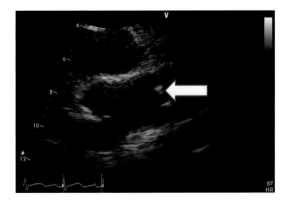

    A. Vegetation
    B. Prosthetic valve
    C. Aortic dissection
    D. Possibly an artifact but need additional views

14. This subcostal image shows:

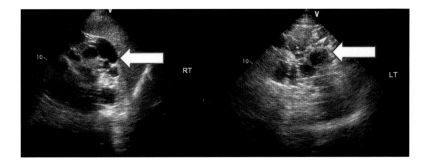

    A. Normal liver
    B. Normal kidney
    C. Cysts in the kidney
    D. Cysts in the liver

15. A 74-year-old male was seen in the emergency room for complaints of severe chest pain. Transthoracic images were suboptimal and a transesophageal echocardiogram (TEE) was ordered. The image shows:

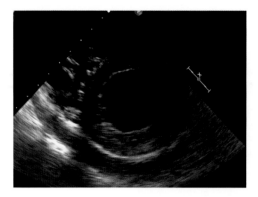

A. Pleural effusion
B. Pericardial effusion
C. Rupture of septum
D. Normal heart

16. This is a mid-esophageal view from the patient in Question 15. The most likely diagnosis is:

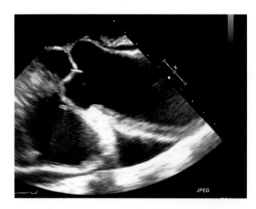

A. Aortic rupture
B. Dissection
C. Artifact
D. None of the above

17. The origin of the dissection is from:

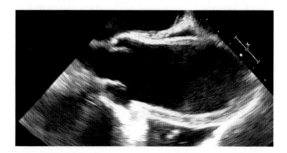

A. Above the left coronary cusp
B. Above the right coronary cusp
C. Above the noncoronary cusp
D. None of the above

18. The best management for the patient in Questions 16–17 is:

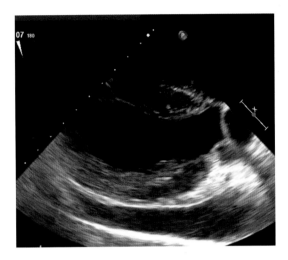

A. Emergency pericardiocentesis
B. Emergency surgery to replace ascending aorta
C. Medical management
D. None of the above

19. The structure pointed to by the arrow is:

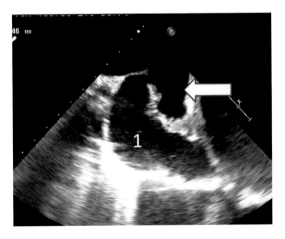

A. Right ventricle (RV)
B. Left atrium (LA)
C. RA appendage
D. LV

20. A 32-year-old female has a history of systemic lupus erythematosus (SLE). She was admitted with complaints of severe shortness of breath. A systolic frame of a four-chamber view shows:

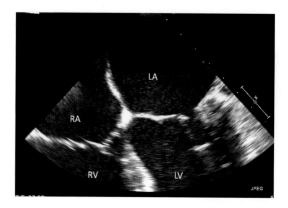

A. Libman Sach's endocarditis
B. Bacterial endocarditis
C. Post-inflammatory changes of the mitral valve
D. Normal mitral valve

Answers for Chapter 23

1. **Answer: C.**
   This is a short axis view of the heart. The image shows underfilled cardiac chambers (LV and RV) surrounded by a large pericardial effusion.

2. **Answer: B.**
   The arrow points to diastolic RV collapse. The RV anterior wall is the anterior-most structure. This is suggestive of pericardial tamponade. Also note that in the 2D reference image the posterior pericardia effusion tracks anterior to the descending aorta. Pleural effusion would track posterior to the aorta.

3. **Answer: B.**
   The Doppler flow pattern across the aortic valve shows marked respirophasic variation (> 25%) in flow, which is a sign of ventricular interdependence and tamponade physiology.

4. **Answer: D.**
   The flow pattern shows ventricular interdependence. The difference between the inspiratory and expiratory velocities should be more than 40% to be specific for tamponade.

5. **Answer. C.**
   The dilated IVC is suggestive of high RA pressure. The presence of pericardial effusion, diastolic RV collapse, ventricular dependence, and elevated RA pressure is suggestive of tamponade.

6. **Answer: C.**
   This is an apical view, showing a large pericardial effusion and a catheter in the pericardial space. Echoguidance during pericardiocentesis allows selection of the most suitable approach and safe entry into the pericardial space. Apical approach is most suitable in > 90% of patients.

7. **Answer: B.**
   This is a subcostal image showing a large left pleural effusion.

8. **Answer: B.**
   The image shows recurrence of pericardial effusion. The arrow points to a mass in the pericardial space. The pericardial fluid analysis showed metastasis from breast cancer.

9. **Answer: B.**
   The presence of reduced systolic function, pericardial effusion, and high eosinophilic count point toward eosinophilic myocarditis. Eosinophilic myocarditis is a rare disorder, often discovered post mortem: 0.5% autopsy series, 20% explanted hearts. Numerous causes include parasitic, idiopathic, drug hypersensitivity, vasculitis-like Churg-Strauss, acute necrotizing, and unknown etiology. Cardiac disease can occur in 50% of idiopathic cases (absolute eosinophilic count $1.5 \times 109/L$). Myocardial infiltrate, perivascular or interstitial, associated with necrosis is seen. Diagnostic tests include echo, cardiovascular magnetic resonance imaging (CMR), biopsy, and bone marrow biopsy. Steroids, immunosuppressive therapy, inotropes, and circulatory support are the mainstay of therapy.

10. **Answer: D.**
    The image shows a complete AV canal defect. Note the defects in the primum atrial septum, inflow part of ventricular septum, and common AV valve.

11. **Answer: B.**
    There is a right to left shunt as demonstrated in the figure. The saline bubbles appeared on the left side after 13 beats, which is suggestive of transpulmonary shunt. Shunting across an PFO or atrial septal defect usually arrives in the LA within four beats.

12. **Answer: C.**
    Flow in the left coronary artery seen from a parasternal short axis view.

13. **Answer: D.**
    A short axis view of the ascending aorta was useful to show that it was an artifact that went through the aortic wall.

14. **Answer: C.**
    These images are obtained from a subcostal view. The left panel shows normal liver tissue and a polycystic right kidney. The right panel shows a polycystic left kidney.

15. **Answer: B.**
    Pericardial effusion is seen in this transgastric image. Since the patient is complaining of chest pain, further imaging is warranted to ascertain the cause.

16. **Answer: B.**
    There is dissection in the aorta with a flap on the anterior wall (greater curvature of aorta) of the ascending aorta.

17. **Answer: B.**
    The tear starts in the aorta just above the origin of the right coronary artery.

18. **Answer: B.**
    This patient has Stanford type A dissection. The patient has a pericardial effusion related to the tear in the aorta and is leaking into the pericardial space. The best management is to transfer the patient to the OR urgently. Pericardiocentesis is contraindicated in this situation. One should not attempt to perform coronary angiogram or aortogram.

19. **Answer: B.**
    The arrow points to the RA appendage. This is a mid-esophageal view with clock-wise rotation. There is associated pericardial effusion denoted by no. 1.

20. **Answer: C.**
    The systolic frame of the four-chamber view shows an enlarged LA. There is a cooptation defect in the mitral valve. The mitral valve shows no evidence of either bacterial or nonbacterial endocarditis. Because the patient has a history of SLE, the mitral valve probably was involved in inflammation that destroyed the valve, leading to a cooptation defect and severe mitral regurgitation.

24

Questions

1. A two-chamber view (systolic frame) of the patient in Chapter 23, Question 20. LA, left atrium. The arrow points to a defect in:

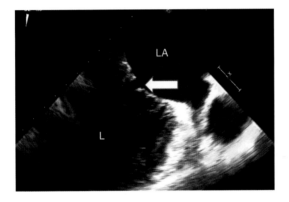

   A. P1 scallop
   B. P2, A2 scallops
   C. P3 scallops
   D. A3 scallop

Echocardiography Board Review: 600 Multiple Choice Questions with Discussion, Third Edition.
Ramdas G. Pai and Padmini Varadarajan.
© 2025 John Wiley & Sons Ltd. Published 2025 by John Wiley & Sons Ltd.

2. The transesophageal echocardiogram (TEE) image of the same patient shows:

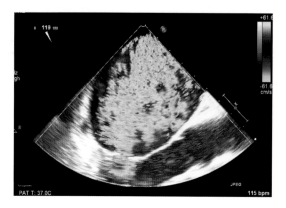

A. Severe mitral regurgitation (MR)
B. 2+ MR
C. Severe tricuspid regurgitation (TR)
D. None of the above

3. This pulse Doppler signal from a TEE image from the same patient is suggestive of:

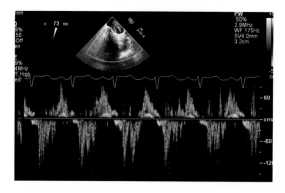

A. Normal pattern of pulmonary vein pattern
B. Systolic flow reversal in the pulmonary vein suggestive of severe MR
C. Systolic flow reversal in the superior vena cava (SVC) suggestive of severe TR
D. None of the above

4. This is a TEE image from the mid-esophageal position of the same patient. The arrow points to:

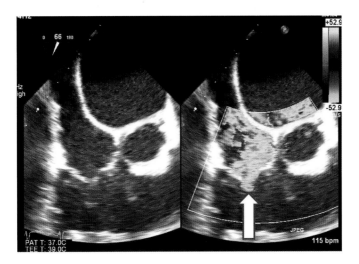

   A. Mild TR
   B. Moderate TR
   C. Severe TR
   D. None of the above

5. The continuous wave pattern from the same patient (right atrial (RA) pressure was 20 mmHg) is suggestive of:

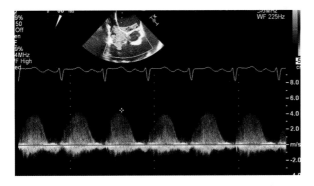

   A. Severe pulmonary hypertension
   B. Moderate pulmonary hypertension
   C. Mild pulmonary hypertension
   D. Cannot be determined

6. This is a TEE image of a four-chamber view from a 32-year-old male patient. The abnormality noted is:

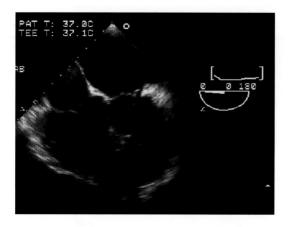

    A. Dextro-transposition of the great arteries (D-TGA)
    B. Levo-transposition of the great arteries (L-TGA)
    C. Dextrocardia
    D. Normal heart

7. The numbers 1 and 2 depict these structures:

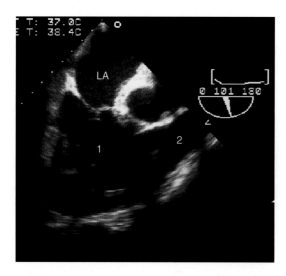

    A. Morphological left ventricle (LV) and aorta
    B. Morphological LV and pulmonary artery (PV)

    C. Morphological right ventricle (RV) and pulmonary artery (PA)

    D. Morphological RV and aorta

8. The numbers 1 and 2 denote:

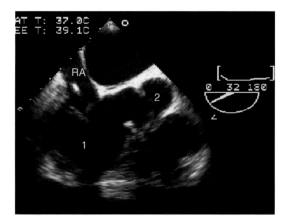

    A. Morphological LV and aorta

    B. Morphological LV and PA

    C. Morphological RV and PA

    D. Morphological RV and aorta

9. The numbers 1 and 2 denote these structures:

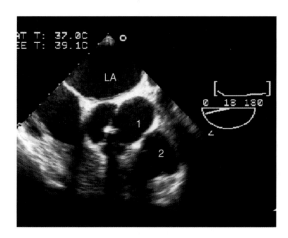

    A. Aortic valve, pulmonary valve

    B. Short axis of mitral, tricuspid valves

    C. Pulmonary valve, aortic valve

    D. None of the above

10. The diastolic and systolic frames of the pulmonary valve flow are suggestive of:

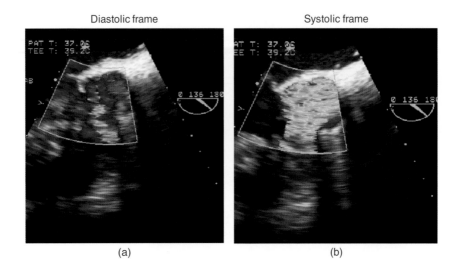

Diastolic frame   Systolic frame

(a)   (b)

A. Mild pulmonary regurgitation (PR) only
B. Mild PR, moderate to severe pulmonary stenosis (PS)
C. Normal flow pattern
D. Cannot be determined

11. This is a parasternal long axis view from a 28-year-old female complaining of shortness of breath. She gives a history of "heart surgery" as a child. The image is suggestive of:

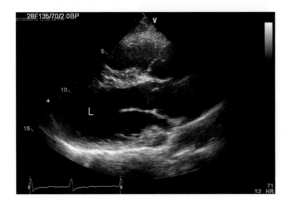

A. Normal chamber orientation
B. D-TGA
C. L-TGA
D. Cannot determine

12. This is a still frame of an apical view. The arrow points to:

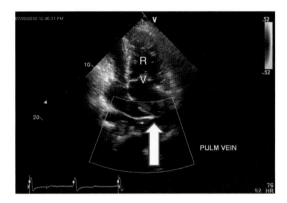

    A. Pulmonary vein
    B. SVC
    C. Inferior vena cava (IVC)
    D. Pulmonary vein baffle into RA

13. This is a still frame of an apical view. The arrow depicts:

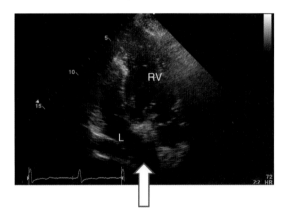

    A. IVC
    B. Pulmonary veins
    C. PA
    D. Systemic venous baffle into LA

14. This is an echo image from a 23-year-old female complaining of shortness of breath. She has a history of D-TGA following a Mustard procedure. Saline contrast was injected from the arm. The image is suggestive of:

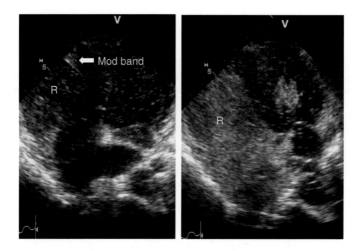

A. Normal saline contrast image
B. Baffle leak
C. Baffle obstruction
D. Need more information

15. This is a parasternal long axis view from a patient with D-TGA following a Mustard procedure. The arrow points to:

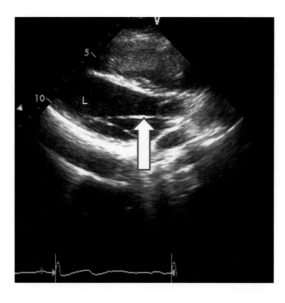

A. False tendon
B. Papillary muscle
C. Pacemaker lead
D. Artifact

16. A 40-year-old male, previously an athlete, was referred for an echocardiogram for complaints of severe shortness of breath. On the basis of the parasternal long axis image of the heart and ECG, you suspect:

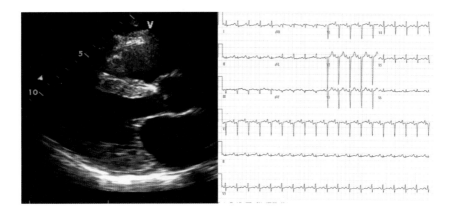

A. Normal LV
B. Hypertrophic cardiomyopathy
C. Amyloidosis
D. Pericarditis

17. A 70-year-old female with a history of Hodgkin's lymphoma and of radiation therapy had an echocardiogram for complaints of shortness of breath. The parasternal long and short axis images are suggestive of:

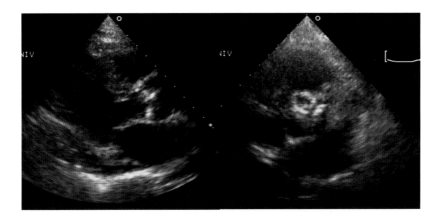

   A. Normal valves

   B. Radiation-induced aortic valve calcification

   C. Endocarditis of the aortic valve

   D. Rheumatic changes of the aortic valve

18. A 30-year-old female with a history of systemic lupus erythematosus (SLE) was admitted with complaints of fever, malaise, chills, and shortness of breath. The still frame of the parasternal long axis image is suggestive of:

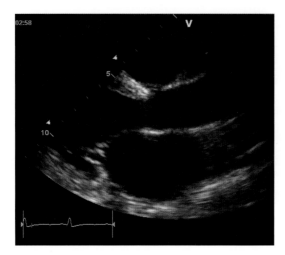

   A. Libman-Sach's endocarditis of the mitral valve

   B. Normal mitral valve

   C. Endocarditis of the aortic valve

   D. Cannot be determined

19. A 58-year-old female with a history of cardiomyopathy and of ventricular tachycardia had this echocardiogram. The accompanying magnetic resonance image (MRI) is shown. The images are suggestive of:

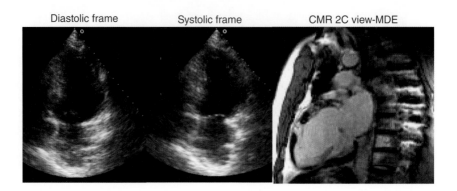

Diastolic frame   Systolic frame   CMR 2C view-MDE

   A. Coronary artery disease

   B. Sarcoidosis

C. Myocarditis

D. None of the above

20. A 44-year-old male with lupus nephritis had complaints of fatigue, malaise, and fever. The patient was on hemodialysis through a temporary subclavian line. The still frame of a long axis view of the heart from a TEE is suggestive of:

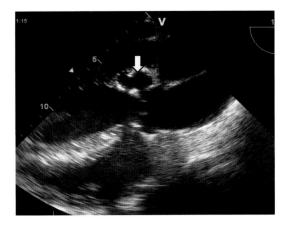

A. Calcified aortic and mitral valves

B. Abscess involving mitral-aortic intervalvular fibrosa

C. Normal valves

D. Bioprosthetic valves

Answers for Chapter 24

1. **Answer: B.**
   This is a TEE image of a commissural view. There is a defect in the mitral valve in the middle, where P2 or A2 scallops would be. These scallops were probably inflamed leading to destruction.

2. **Answer: A.**
   The TEE image (long axis) shows color filling the entire left atrium. The origin of the jet is at P2/A2 scallops, where the valve leaflets have been destroyed. The proximal isovelocity surface area (PISA) is large, which is suggestive of a large volume of regurgitation.

3. **Answer. B.**
   The pulse wave Doppler pattern was obtained from the right upper pulmonary vein. The pulse wave Doppler shows systolic flow reversal. This is indicative of severe MR and is another sign that can be coupled with color flow imaging to evaluate for severity of MR.

4. **Answer: C.**
   The TEE image is obtained by clockwise rotation from the mid esophagus. This helps in visualization of the tricuspid valve. The color flow imaging shows the TR jet with a vena contracta diameter of 8 mm suggestive of severe TR.

5. **Answer: A.**
   This patient's TR velocity was measured at 4.5 m/s. This yields an RA–RV gradient of 81 mmHg. With a RA pressure of 20, her RV systolic pressure was 100 mmHg, which is suggestive of severe pulmonary hypertension.

6. **Answer: B.**
   The left-sided ventricle that is in continuity with LA has an atrioventricular valve that is closer to the apex, suggestive of morphologic RV. The right-sided ventricle is the morphologic LV with mitral valve. The RA is connected to the LV and the LA is connected to the RV. There is ventriculo-atrial discordance.

7. **Answer: D.**
   This TEE image shows the morphologic RV connected to the transposed aorta, which lies to the left of the pulmonary artery. There is heavy trabeculation (arrow), which also helps is identifying this chamber as the morphologic RV, which also goes with the tricuspid valve.

8. **Answer: B.**
   This image shows the morphologic LV connected to the PA. The chamber is smoother with fewer trabeculations suggestive of morphologic LV. In this image the left-sided aorta is also seen. The RA is connected to the LV. Thus, there is atrio-ventricular and ventriculo-arterial discordance, two wrongs making it "right." This is suggestive of congenitally corrected transposition or L-TGA.

9. **Answer: C.**
   This is a TEE short axis image at the basal level. Both the great vessels are seen in short axis as opposed to the normal depiction of one great vessel (usually the aorta) in short axis and the pulmonary artery in long axis. Both the valves are

seen in short axis orientation, which is pathognomonic for transposition. The pulmonary valve is also thickened. This should be recognized as transposition of great vessels.

10. **Answer B.**
These images show color flow images of the pulmonary valve – the diastolic frame revealing mild PR (panel A) and the systolic frame showing aliasing and turbulence suggestive of pulmonary stenosis (panel B).

11. **Answer: B.**
D-transposition. This is a transthoracic image from a parasternal long axis view of the heart. The most noticeable feature is the depiction of both great arteries in parallel. This is very characteristic of transposition of great arteries. Normally only the aorta is visible in the parasternal long axis view. In the parasternal short axis view both arteries are visible, the aorta in short axis and the pulmonary artery in long axis. In D-TGA the aorta is anterior and is connected to the trabeculated RV. The PA is connected to the LV. Here, the LV is connected to a posteriorly situated great vessel, the PA.

12. **Answer: D.**
This is an apical four-chamber view of the heart. Because the patient had undergone surgical correction with the Mustard procedure, the pulmonary veins are baffled into the RA and the systemic veins are baffled into the LA. The white arrow points to the pulmonary venous baffle.

13. **Answer D.**
This is an apical four-chamber view of the heart. The white arrow points to the systemic venous baffle.

14. **Answer: B.**
A saline contrast echocardiogram performed from the arm showed dense opacification of the systemic RV, suggesting a massive baffle leak from right to left causing hypoxemia. Also note the moderator band in the RV.

15. **Answer: C.**
This is a parasternal long axis view showing a pacer lead in the LV, which is the subpulmonic ventricle or the venous ventricle.

16. **Answer: C.**
This figure shows a parasternal long axis view of the heart. There is LV hypertrophy. There is a sparkling appearance to the myocardium. The figure also shows a 12-lead ECG of the patient. There is low voltage in all the limb leads. The combination of LV hypertrophy on echo and low voltage on ECG is suggestive of an infiltrative disease such as amyloid.

17. **Answer: B.**
The still frame is a parasternal long axis view of the heart. The valve is severely calcified and is not opening well (systolic frame of the short axis image). The aortic valve is severely stenosed, which is an effect of prior radiation therapy. Radiation-induced carditis can be associated with pericardial thickening leading to constrictive pericarditis. Associated calcific stenosis of the aortic and mitral valves is commonly seen. Some patients can also have calcific stenosis of the coronary arteries.

18. **Answer: A.**

    This is a still frame of a parasternal long axis image. There is a small mass attached to the posterior mitral leaflet suggestive of Libman-Sach's, which is a common finding in SLE.

19. **Answer: B.**

    This is a still frame of her two-chamber view. There is a localized aneurysm in the mid-anterior wall. The patient was worked up for sarcoidosis. The accompanying cardiac magnetic resonance (CMR) image shows a transmural scar in the mid-anterior wall (the bright area denotes scar). The scar distribution in sarcoidosis is typically in the lateral wall and is mostly epicardial. There can also be a mid-myocardial scar and a scar in the RV.

20. **Answer: B.**

    This is a long axis view (TEE) from a mid-esophageal level from the patient described in Question 19. The aortic valve is thickened. There is an echo-free space (arrow) adjacent to the aortic valve suggestive of an abscess of the fibrous continuity of the aortic and mitral valves (mitral intervalvular fibrosa). This patient had lupus nephritis. His aortic valve probably started out with endocarditis, which in due course progressed to an abscess.

25

Questions

1. This still-frame image of a four-chamber view shows:

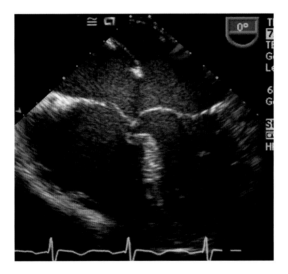

   A. Secundum atrial septal defect (ASD)
   B. Primum ASD
   C. Sinus venosus ASD
   D. None of the above

Echocardiography Board Review: 600 Multiple Choice Questions with Discussion, Third Edition.
Ramdas G. Pai and Padmini Varadarajan.
© 2025 John Wiley & Sons Ltd. Published 2025 by John Wiley & Sons Ltd.

2. LV, left ventricle. The still-frame image of an apical five-chamber view shows:

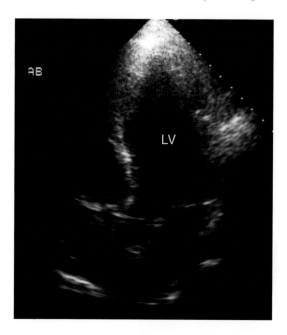

A. Artifact
B. Anomalous coronary artery
C. Coronary sinus
D. Biventricular pacer lead

3. AV, aortic valve; RVOT, right ventricular outflow tract. This parasternal short axis view shows:

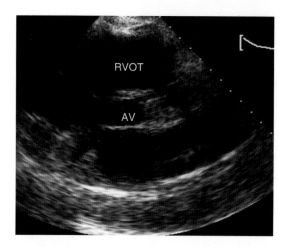

A. Normal aorta and pulmonary artery
B. Imaging artifact

    C. Anomalous coronary artery

    D. Artifact from pulmonary prosthesis

4. This 51-year-old Armenian male was admitted with complaints of chest pain. He underwent an echocardiogram. The still frame of 2D and color image show:

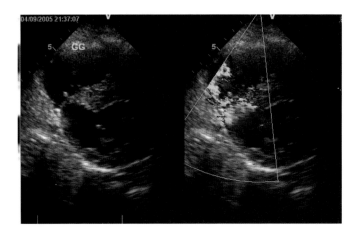

    A. ASD

    B. Inferior septal ventricular septal defect (VSD)

    C. Muscular VSD

    D. None of the above

5. The continuous wave Doppler shows:

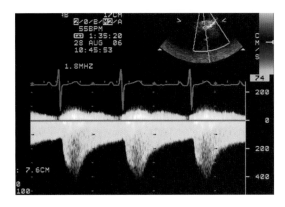

    A. Patent ductus arteriosus (PDA)

    B. Coarctation of the aorta

    C. Coronary fistula

    D. None of the above

6. This still-frame image of a subcostal view shows:

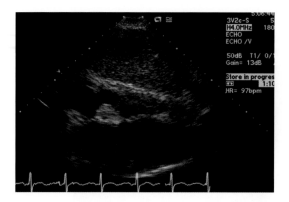

  A. Myxoma
  B. Lipoma
  C. Lipomatous hypertrophy of the interatrial septum
  D. Thrombus attached to the interatrial septum

7. This still frame of a color flow four-chamber view shows:

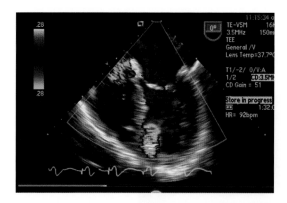

  A. Muscular VSD
  B. Apical cannula flow of a left ventricular assist device (LVAD)
  C. Pseudoaneurysm
  D. None of the above

8. The color flow obtained from parasternal short axis and suprasternal views shows:

Parasternal short axis view   Suprasternal view

A. Pulmonary regurgitation
B. PDA
C. Coronary fistula
D. Flow in the coronary artery

9. A 41-year-old male complained of diarrhea, flushing, and weight loss. This image
   obtained from the subcostal view shows:

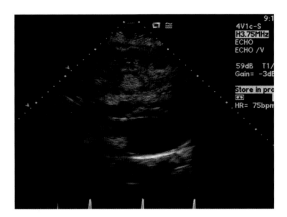

A. Normal heart and liver
B. Carcinoid masses in the liver
C. Liver cysts
D. None of the above

10. This still-frame image of an apical long axis view shows:

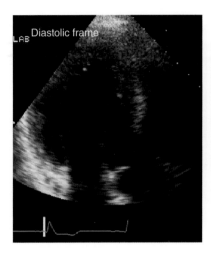 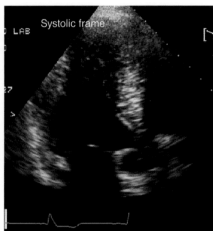

   A. Normal appearance of the heart
   B. Hypertrophy of the septum
   C. Apical hypertrophic cardiomyopathy
   D. Apical thrombus

11. This is a 40-year-old male with a history of Marfan syndrome. The still-frame image of a parasternal short axis and parasternal long axis view shows this surgical procedure that the patient has undergone:

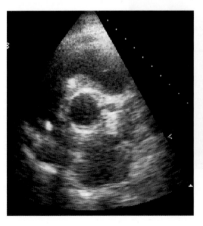 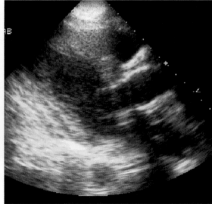

   A. Coronary artery bypass
   B. Bentall
   C. Ascending aortic graft
   D. None of the above

12. A 22-year-old male had an echocardiogram as part of routine surveillance. The short axis image shows:

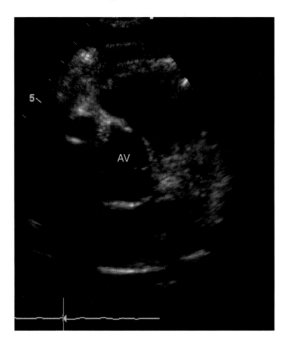

A. Anomalous coronary artery
B. Aneurysmal dilatation of the right coronary artery
C. Sinus of Valsalva aneurysm
D. None of the above

13. A 38-year-old male complained of fever, chills, and weight loss. The 2D and color flow of the parasternal long axis images show:

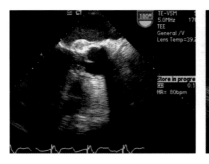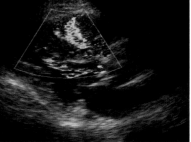

A. Vegetation of the aortic valve
B. Abscess involving the aortic valve with fistula into the right ventricle
C. Vegetation of the mitral valve
D. None of the above

14. A 21-year-old male with a history of heart transplant had this echocardiogram. The short-axis and four-chamber color flow show:

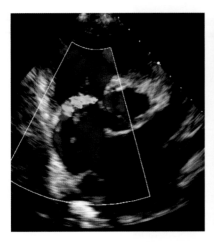 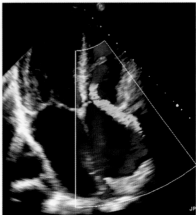

    A. Mild tricuspid regurgitation (TR)
    B. Moderate TR
    C. Severe TR
    D. None of the above

15. The Doppler flow is suggestive of:

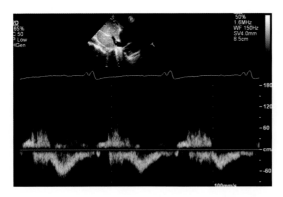

    A. Normal hepatic flow
    B. Severe TR
    C. Cardiac tamponade
    D. Constrictive pericarditis

16. The subcostal image shows:

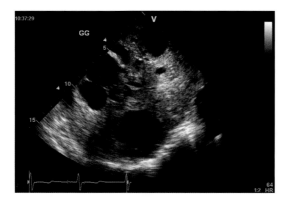

   A. Normal appearance of the liver
   B. Multiple cysts of the liver
   C. Multiple tumors in the liver
   D. None of the above

17. The continuous wave Doppler flow is suggestive of:

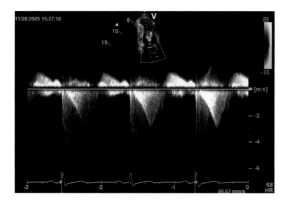

   A. Severe mitral regurgitation
   B. Left ventricular (LV) mid-cavity obliteration
   C. Dynamic outflow obstruction
   D. Severe aortic stenosis

18. The apical four-chamber and subcostal views show:

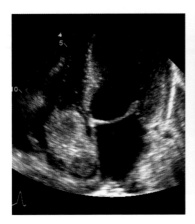 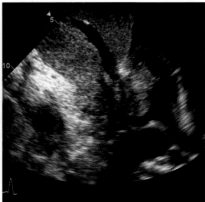

   A. Thrombus in the right atrium (RA)
   B. Tumor invasion of the RA through the inferior vena cava (IVC)
   C. Myxoma of the RA
   D. Lipomatous hypertrophy of the atrial septum

19. The subcostal view shows:

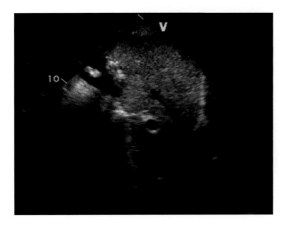

   A. Normal liver and gall bladder
   B. Gall stones
   C. Cysts in the liver
   D. Tumor of the liver

20. A 55-year-old male complained of shortness of breath and pedal edema, progressively worsening for 2 months. He had an echocardiogram. Representative four-chamber and short axis views show:

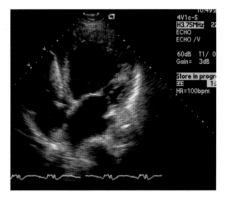 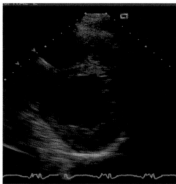

A. Normal LV
B. Apical hypertrophic cardiomyopathy
C. Noncompaction of LV
D. Apical ballooning

Answers for Chapter 25

1. **Answer: B.**
   The still-frame image shows a defect in the lower portion of the atrial septum. This constitutes a primum ASD. Often this is associated with a cleft in the mitral valve. This is also known as a partial atrioventricular canal defect.

2. **Answer: B.**
   The still frame shows a tubular structure crossing the ascending aorta. This is an anomalous coronary artery.

3. **Answer: C.**
   The parasternal short axis image shows a tubular structure crossing from the right coronary cusp to the left side. This is an anomalous left anterior descending artery arising from the right coronary cusp.

4. **Answer: B.**
   This patient who came with chest pain had an inferior myocardial infarction (MI). The 2D image shows a defect in the inferior septum. The accompanying color flow image shows a left to side shunt across the inferior septum. This is a common mechanical complication to look for in patients with an inferior MI.

5. **Answer: B.**
   This is a continuous wave Doppler obtained from the suprasternal view. There is a prominent systolic component with a peak velocity of 4 m/s, along with diastolic flow. This typical saw tooth pattern is seen in coarctation of aorta with significant stenosis.

6. **Answer: C.**
   This is a still-frame four-chamber view obtained from the subcostal view. The interatrial septum appears like a dumb bell with a thin fossa ovalis in the center. This is a typical appearance of lipomatuos interatrial septum.

7. **Answer: B.**
   The color flow image was obtained from the apical view. There is color flow seen at the apex. This represents flow through the apical inlet cannula of an LVAD.

8. **Answer: B.**
   The still frame of the parasternal short axis view shows color flow in the pulmonary artery. The accompanying suprasternal view shows flow from the aorta into the left pulmonary artery. This is representative of PDA.

9. **Answer: B.**
   This subcostal image shows hyperechoic masses in the liver. These patients with complaints of flushing, diarrhea, and weight loss are representative of carcinoid disease.

10. **Answer: C.**
    The still frame of diastolic and systolic frame of the LV shows a thickened apex. The apex is usually a thin structure. Here the apex measures about 1 cm in diastole. This demonstrates apical hypertrophy of the LV.

11. **Answer: B.**
    The long axis image shows a tube-like structure inside the aorta. This patient has undergone a Bentall procedure, which is a composite of an ascending tube graft and a prosthetic valve. The coronary arteries were also reimplanted.

12. **Answer: C.**
    This patient's echocardiogram reveals a dilated and aneurysmal right coronary artery. This is a result of Kawasaki disease. The disease causes inflammation in the walls of small and medium-sized arteries including the coronary arteries. It is also known as mucocutaneous lymph node syndrome as it affects lymph nodes and mucous membranes of nose, mouth, and throat. An echocardiogram typically shows aneurysmal dilatation of the coronary arteries.

13. **Answer: B.**
    The 2D image shows a hypoechoic structure involving the aortic valve. This bulging structure represents an abscess due to endocarditis. The color flow image shows a fistulous communication into the RV, which is due to the abscess rupturing into the RV.

14. **Answer: C.**
    The color flow images show an eccentric TR. The color flow is suggestive of severe TR. The color flow of TR is directed away from the septal leaflet. The eccentricity of the jet is suggestive of a probable flail of the septal leaflet. This could be due to multiple biopsies that these patients undergo.

15. **Answer: B.**
    The Doppler flow was obtained from the hepatic vein from the patient in Question 494. There is systolic flow reversal that is suggestive of severe TR.

16. **Answer: B.**
    The subcostal view of the liver shows multiple septations with hypoechoic areas. These hypoechoic areas are simple cysts of the liver. These occur in patients with polycystic disease, usually of the kidney and liver.

17. **Answer: B.**
    The continuous flow Doppler is obtained from the apical view. There is evidence of MR flow (faint signal). Superimposed on and within this signal there is a late peaking, dagger-shaped systolic flow. This is due to mid-cavity obliteration.

18. **Answer: B.**
    There is a mass visible in the right atrium. The subcostal view shows tumor masses in the IVC, with direct extension into the RA.

19. **Answer: B.**
    The image shows dense structures in the gall bladder. There is shadowing across the gall bladder arising from these structures.

20. **Answer: C.**
    The echocardiogram shows noncompaction of the LV. The lateral wall is heavily trabeculated. Noncompaction by echo can be diagnosed when the ratio of non-compacted myocardium to compacted myocardium is greater than 2 in diastole.

26

Questions

1. A 20-year-old male presented with shortness of breath, large right ventricle (RV) and right atrium (RA), and pulmonary artery (PA) systolic pressure of 30 mmHg. The image shows:

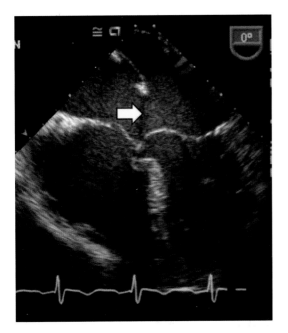

    A. Ostium primum atrial septal defect (ASD)
    B. Sinus venosus ASD of inferior vena cava (IVC) type
    C. Sinus venosus of superior vena cava (SVC) type
    D. Secundum ASD

Echocardiography Board Review: 600 Multiple Choice Questions with Discussion, Third Edition.
Ramdas G. Pai and Padmini Varadarajan.
© 2025 John Wiley & Sons Ltd. Published 2025 by John Wiley & Sons Ltd.

2. In the patient in Question 1, the most commonly seen associated defect would be:
   A. Ventricular septal defect (VSD)
   B. Coarctation of the aorta
   C. Bicuspid aortic valve
   D. Cleft of the anterior mitral leaflet

3. The echocardiographic image of the patient in Question 1 shows a dilated RV and RA with a PA pressure of 30 mmHg. The recommended definitive treatment for this patient would be:
   A. Annual follow-up
   B. Percutaneous closure of the defect
   C. Surgical closure of the defect
   D. Medical management

4. Tetralogy of Fallot may be associated with this genetic mutation:
   A. Point mutation in the major histocompatibility complex gene
   B. 22q11 deletion
   C. 9–22 translocation
   D. Trisomy of chromosome 21

5. The continuous wave Doppler in the image obtained from the suprasternal window is indicative of:

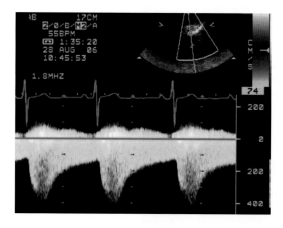

   A. Patent ductus arteriosus (PDA)
   B. Coarctation of the aorta
   C. Coronary artery fistula
   D. Coronary stenosis

6. Endocarditis prophylaxis in indicated in all patients with adult congenital heart disease except:
   A. Those with a previous history of endocarditis
   B. Patients with placement of prosthetic material after 12 months
   C. Patients with uncorrected cyanotic heart disease
   D. Patients with surgical or transcatheter valves

7. LV, left ventricle. This is true about this patient:

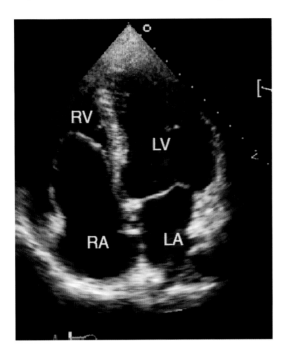

A. Patient may have severe tricuspid regurgitation and heart failure
B. Patient may be cyanotic
C. Patient may present with atrial arrhythmias and reentrant arrhythmias due to accessory pathways
D. All of the above
E. None of the above.

8. A patient had surgery for cyanotic heart disease as a child. The continuous wave Doppler signal from the pulmonary valve is shown in this image. This patient is likely to have had this condition as a child for which surgery was undertaken:

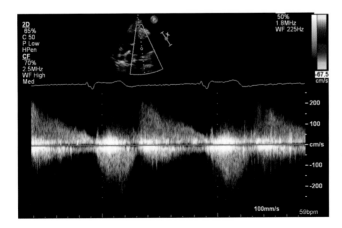

   A. Tetralogy of Fallot
   B. Transposition of great vessels
   C. Tricuspid atresia
   D. Total anomalous pulmonary venous drainage

9. A, aorta; DC, distal chamber; PC, proximal chamber. A 40-year-old male patient is referred for an echocardiogram. This image shows:

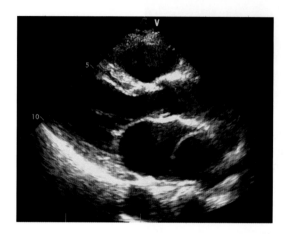

   A. Supravalvular mitral ring
   B. Cor triatriatum sinister
   C. Cor triatriatum dexter
   D. Left atrial cyst

10. A 22-year-old male is referred to your clinic with symptoms of dyspnea on exertion. A year ago the patient was being evaluated for similar complaints. Further evaluation of the patient with an echocardiogram showed cor triatriatum sinister with a gradient of 10 mmHg. The patient was referred to surgery and had the membrane resected. The patient felt better soon after the surgery, but a few months later started noticing dyspnea. In this patient you would suspect:
   A. Recurrence of cor triatriatum
   B. Pulmonary vein stenosis
   C. Mitral stenosis
   D. ASD
   E. None of the above

11. A 30-year-old male is referred to your clinic for a consult for evaluation of murmur. He gives a history of recent dyspnea on exertion. Examination reveals heart rate of 75/min, BP 129/76 mmHg, mildly elevated jugular venous pressure, and systolic murmur at the second right intercostal space. He then undergoes an echocardiogram that reveals normal LV size and severe concentric LV hypertrophy with an ejection fraction of 60%. Mitral valve shows mild mitral and aortic regurgitation. The murmur is due to:

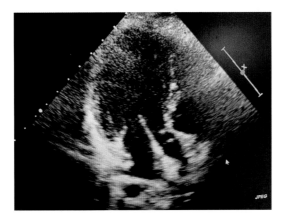

A. Mitral stenosis

B. Rheumatic aortic valve disease

C. Subaortic membrane

D. Supraaortic membrane

12. A 32-year-old male is referred to your clinic for evaluation of murmur. He gives a history of recent dyspnea on exertion. Examination reveals heart rate of 80/min, BP 121/70 mmHg, mildly elevated jugular venous pressure, and systolic murmur at the second right intercostal space. He then undergoes an echocardiogram that reveals normal LV size and severe concentric LV hypertrophy with an ejection fraction of 45%. Aortic valve is trileaflet and opens well with no evidence of stenosis. Doppler evaluation shows flow acceleration below the aortic valve, peak velocity is 3.7 m/sec, peak gradient of 55 mmHg. Careful evaluation then shows a discrete membrane just below the aortic valve. Mitral valve shows mild mitral and aortic regurgitation. The best management strategy in this patient is:

A. Repeat echocardiogram in 3 months

B. Repeat echocardiogram in 6 months

C. Surgical resection of the subaortic membrane

D. Medical management

13. A 27-year-old male is referred to your clinic with complains of chest pain. On further questioning, the patient complains of chest pain, characterized as a pressure-like feeling, exacerbated with exertion and relieved with rest. He does not have any significant past history or family history. On examination vital signs are stable. Cardiac exam is within normal limits. He then undergoes an echocardiogram. His images are difficult. Since he was symptomatic, he underwent coronary CT angiogram that shows anomalous origin of the right coronary artery from the left coronary sinus. The next best step is:

A. Nothing to do at this time

B. Stress test to evaluate for ischemia

C. Coronary angiogram

D. Medical therapy for chest pain

14. The patient in this image has this condition:

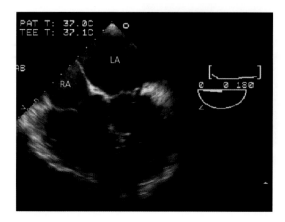

    A. Congenitally corrected transposition of the great arteries (L-TGA)
    B. Transposition of the great arteries (D-TGA)
    C. Ebstein's anomaly
    D. None of the above

15. The patient in this image has this condition:

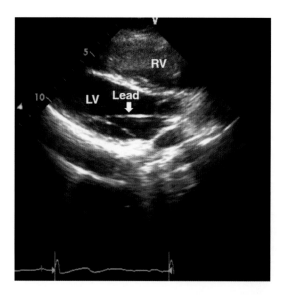

    A. Congenitally corrected transposition of the great vessels
    B. D-TGA with atrial switch
    C. D-TGA with arterial switch
    D. None of the above

16. A 21-year-old male comes for evaluation of palpitations. He was diagnosed with congenital heart disease during his childhood. History included exposure to drugs by his mother while pregnant. On the exam he has a noteworthy 3/6 holosystolic murmur

at increases with inspiration at left lower sternal border. Exam unremarkable otherwise. ECG shows evidence of right atrial enlargement and right bundle branch block (RBBB). A still frame of his echo is shown. If his mother was exposed during pregnancy, this medication would be a culprit in causing this congenital lesion:

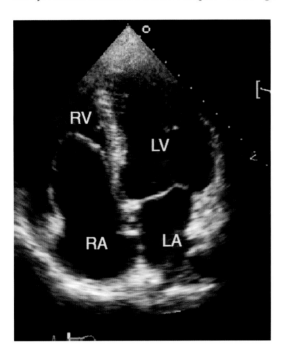

A. Ibuprofen
B. Lithium
C. Metoprolol
D. Angiotensin-converting enzyme (ACE) inhibitor

17. A 21-year-old male came for an evaluation of palpitations and fatigue. He had no significant past medical history and denied substance abuse. The examination was unremarkable. ECG was normal. A still frame of his echo shows:

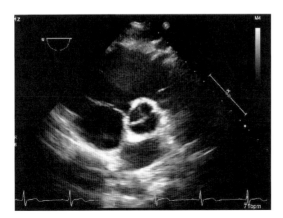

A. Trileaflet aortic valve
B. Pulmonary valve stenosis
C. Bicuspid aortic valve
D. Quadricuspid aortic valve

18. A 40-year-old male was admitted to the hospital for complaints of chest pain. ECG was unremarkable. Exam revealed a 2/4 decrescendo murmur at the second right intercostal space. An echo was performed. This still-frame image shows:

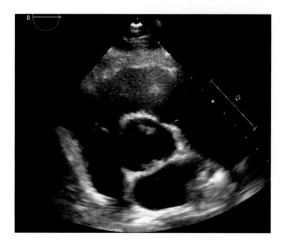

A. Absent pulmonary valve
B. Unicuspid aortic valve
C. Bicuspid aortic valve
D. Subaortic membrane

19. An 18-year-old male is referred for an echocardiogram due to a murmur heard by his primary care physician. On the echocardiogram the patient has mildly dilated left ventricle and left atrium. A small restrictive VSD is visualized. On continuous wave Doppler peak velocity of 5.2 m/sec velocity is obtained. Rest of the examination is normal. His blood pressure during the start of the echocardiogram is 126/70 mmHg. The PA systolic pressure in this patient is:
A. 25 mmHg
B. 18 mmHg
C. 38 mmHg
D. Cannot be estimated

20. A 19-year-old female was referred for an evaluation for ongoing dyspnea. The patient was diagnosed with a congenital heart condition during infancy and underwent a surgical procedure. She was doing fine until a few months ago when she started noticing dyspnea on exertion and fatigue. She is very active and used to be in the cheerleading squad in her high school. This echocardiogram was performed and it shows:

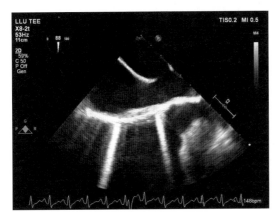

A. Severe pulmonary valve regurgitation
B. Severe PA stenosis
C. Supracristal VSD
D. Patent ductus arteriosus

21. A 30-year-old female was referred for an echocardiogram. A patent foramen ovale is visualized with a systolic velocity of 2.7 m/sec and a diastolic velocity of 0.9 m/sec. Rest of the exam was normal. Assuming RA pressure of 8, what is the estimated LA pressure during systole and diastole?
   A. 37 mmHg during systole and 11 mmHg during diastole
   B. 40 mmHg during systole and 15 mmHg during diastole
   C. 29 mmHg during systole and 3 mmHg during diastole
   D. Cannot be estimated

22. A 20-year-old male was referred for an echocardiogram because of complaints of shortness of breath and fatigue. A still-frame image of transesophageal echocardiogram is shown here. The patient has this lesion:

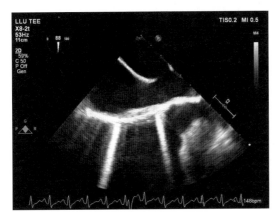

  A. Ostium primum ASD
  B. Ostium secundum ASD
  C. Sinus venosus ASD
  D. VSD

23. A 58-year-old female had an echocardiogram for preoperative evaluation. A still frame of the echocardiogram from an apical view shows this:

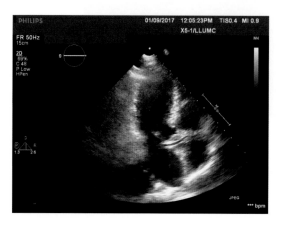

  A. Anomalous right coronary artery from left sinus
  B. Anomalous left circumflex coronary artery from right sinus
  C. Coronary sinus
  D. Pacemaker lead

24. A 20-year-old male student athlete has an echocardiogram for evaluation of murmur. A still frame of the transthoracic echocardiogram (TTE) shows this:

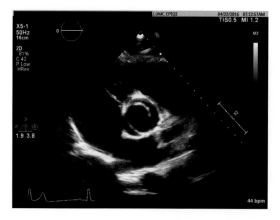

  A. Unicuspid aortic valve
  B. Trileaflet aortic valve
  C. Bicuspid aortic valve with right left fusion
  D. Bicuspid aortic valve with right noncoronary cusp fusion

25. A 14-year-old male was referred for an echocardiogram. In addition to a patent foramen ovale (PFO), the still-frame image from a TTE shows this type of defect:

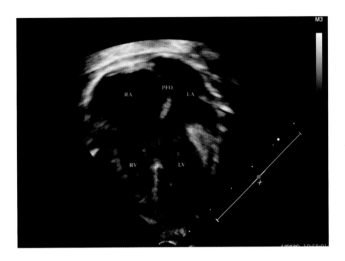

   A. Ostium secundum ASD
   B. Partial atrioventricular (AV) septal defect
   C. VSD
   D. Complete AV septal defect

26. This still-frame image is from a 40-year-old male with a murmur. Color flow Doppler shows a PDA and continuous wave Doppler of the same is also shown. Peak systolic velocity of the continuous flow is 4.7 m/sec. His blood pressure at the time of the study was 118/75 mmHg. LPA/MPA/RPA, left/main/right pulmonary artery; DA, descending aorta. The estimated PA systolic pressure is:

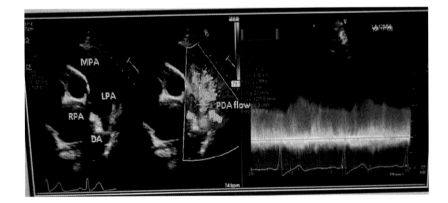

   A. 88 mmHg
   B. 30 mmHg
   C. 98 mmHg
   D. Cannot be estimated

27. This X-ray from an 18-year-old male patient shows this sign:

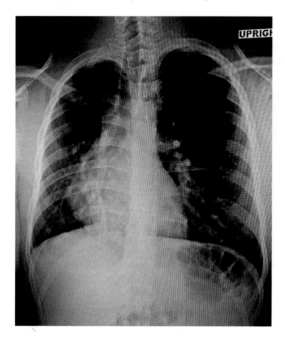

A. Scimitar syndrome
B. Situs inversus
C. Right aortic arch
D. None of the above

28. This still-frame image from the subcostal view is from the patient in Question 27. The image shows:

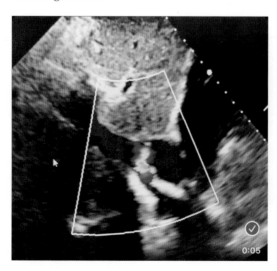

A. Fontan conduit
B. Normal IVC flow

C. Flow from anomalous pulmonary vein into the IVC

D. None of the above

29. This still-frame systolic image from the apical view on a TTE is from a 22-year-old male with a loud holosystolic murmur from the left side of the chest. The echocardiogram shows this lesion:

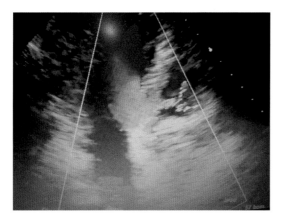

A. Posterior VSD

B. Muscular VSD

C. Supracristal VSD

D. Perimembranous VSD

E. Ruptured sinus of Valsalva

30. This still frame of a continuous wave Doppler waveform was obtained from the ventricular septal flow. Blood pressure at the time of the echocardiogram was 121/65 mmHg. The patient has:

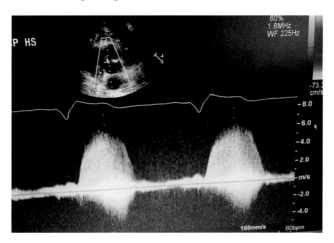

A. Elevated systolic PA pressure

B. Normal systolic PA pressure

C. Low systolic PA pressure

D. Need more information to calculate

E. Cannot be calculated

Answers for Chapter 26

1. **Answer: A.**
   This patient's echocardiographic image shows a defect in the lower part of the atrial septum that constitutes an ostium primum ASD. This is also known as a partial AV canal defect.

2. **Answer: D.**
   The most commonly associated defect seen with a primum ASD is a cleft in the anterior mitral leaflet.

3. **Answer: C.**
   This patient has ostium primum ASD in the lower part of the septum. The patient has volume overload with normal PA pressure and has an indication for closure. This is not amenable to percutaneous closure, unlike a secundum ASD.

4. **Answer: B.**
   Screening for mutations should be offered to all patients with tetralogy of Fallot, who should all, especially those with a heritable mutation, be offered genetic counseling before a planned pregnancy.

5. **Answer: B.**
   Note that the systolic gradient is about 64 mmHg and there is a gradient throughout the diastole. This is indicative of severe aortic coarctation.

6. **Answer: B.**
   The current guideline recommendations for endocarditis prophylaxis includes patients with the following conditions: (1) previous history of endocarditis; (2) within 6 months of placement of prosthetic material for repair; (3) residual shunts at the site of or adjacent to previous repair with prosthetic materials or devices; or (4) uncorrected cyanotic heart disease.

7. **Answer: D.**
   This patient has Ebstein's anomaly with apical displacement of septal tricuspid leaflet and large sail-like anterior leaflet. About 25% have accessory pathways, mostly right, and 50% have patent foramen ovale (PFO) or ASD, facilitating right to left shunting. See the image provided with the question. Note that a large portion of the right ventricle is atrialized.

8. **Answer: A.**
   The image shows Doppler signal suggestive of severe pulmonary regurgitation, which is an important sequela of tetralogy of Fallot repair.

9. **Answer: B.**

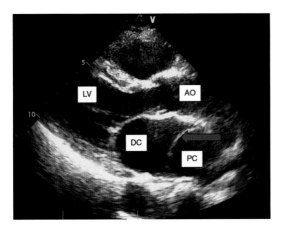

The blue arrow points to a membrane dividing the LA into a proximal chamber (PC) containing the pulmonary veins and a more distal chamber (DC) connected to the mitral valve. This is indicative of cor triatriatum sinister (of LA). A, aorta.

10. **Answer: B.**
In patients who undergo surgery for cor triatriatum and with recurrence of symptoms, pulmonary vein stenosis can occur after surgery. Such patients should undergo evaluation for pulmonary vein stenosis. Pulmonary vein stenosis does not progress over time and has not been associated with pulmonary arterial hypertension.

11. **Answer: C.**

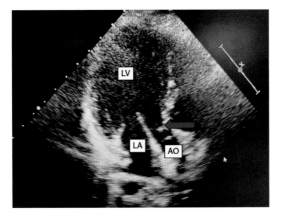

The echo cardiogram shows a subaortic membrane. The arrow in the image points to a structure below the aortic valve that is a subaortic membrane.

12. **Answer: C.**

In patients with subaortic stenosis due to a membrane, surgical resection is recommended (Class 1 C-LD) when gradient is < 50 mmHg, in the presence of heart failure, ischemic symptoms, or LV dysfunction.

Patients with reduced LV function and severe subaortic stenosis may not manifest a gradient of ≥ 50 mmHg. In this subset of patients decisions to cause relief of subaortic stenosis may be extrapolated from aortic stenosis data. In some patients with preserved systolic LV function, compliance may be poor and result in heart failure symptoms and a resting maximum gradient of < 50 mmHg.

Surgical resection in these patients may be beneficial. Patients with resting or stress-induced ischemia in the absence of obstructive coronary artery disease but with moderate subaortic stenosis (maximum gradient > 30 and < 50 mmHg) may benefit from surgical resection.

This patient has a maximum subaortic gradient of 51 mmHg. Surgical resection of the membrane will be beneficial.

13. **Answer: B.**

Stress test In patients with anomalous coronary artery origin. Stress testing should be performed to elicit ischemia, which will dictate further management. Refer to flow chart from 2018 Adult Congenital Heart Diseases guidelines.

14. **Answer: A.**

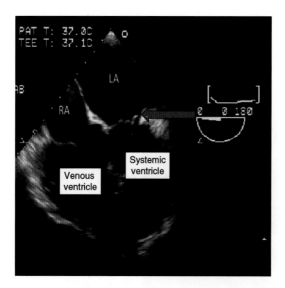

Note that the left AV valve is more apical (blue arrow), indicating that it is the tricuspid valve and the ventricle that goes with it is the RV (systemic ventricle). Hence the mitral valve and morphological LV (venous ventricle) are on the right side. There is AV discordance. This would in addition be associated with ventriculoarterial discordance (RV to aorta and LV to PA), with the two wrongs making a right, and the circulation would be normal except that the systemic ventricle is morphologically the RV and the systemic AV valve is a tricuspid valve. There is a higher risk of tricuspid regurgitation (TR) and RV (systemic ventricle) failure in these patients.

15. **Answer: B.**
    Note the pacer lead in the LV (smooth walled), indicating that it pumps into the pulmonary circulation. This is indicative of atrial switch. In arterial switch the LV would pump into the aorta. In L-TGA or congenitally corrected TGA the posterior ventricle would be a morphological RV, which pumps into the aorta.

16. **Answer: B.**
    The patient has exam findings suggestive of TR. ECG shows right atrial enlargement and RBBB. His echo shows evidence of Ebstein's anomaly. Maternal exposure to lithium and benzodiazepine during pregnancy has been associated with Ebstein's anomaly. Maternal exposure to metoprolol can cause fetal bradycardia and hypoglycemia. ACE inhibitors cause oligohydramnios due to reduced renal function in the fetus, may also lead to fetal lung hypoplasia and skeletal malformations. Ibuprofen has been known to cause constriction of the ductus arteriosus and persistent pulmonary hypertension of the fetus.

17. **Answer: D.**
    The echo image is a still frame of the base of the heart at the level of the aortic valve. The short axis of the aortic valve shows four equal-sized cusps in closed position. This is type A quadricuspid valve. In type B there will be 3 equal cusps and 1 smaller cusp. In type C there will be 2 equal larger cusps and 2 equal smaller cusps. In type D there will be 1 larger cusp, 2 intermediate cusps, and 1 smaller cusp. In type E there will be 3 relatively equal cusps with 1 large cusp. In type F there will be 2 equal large cusps and 2 unequal smaller cusps.

18. **Answer: B.**

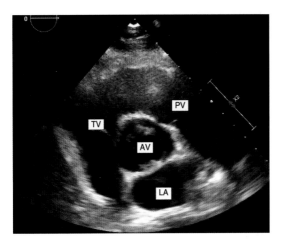

The still frame of the echo is from the base of the heart. It clearly shows a unicuspid valve. The patient also had moderate aortic regurgitation and mild ascending aortic dilatation.

19. **Answer: B.**

   The estimated PA systolic pressure is 18 mmHg. The peak gradient across the VSD is 5.2 m/s, which calculates to a gradient of 108 mmHg (5.2 × 5.2 × 4) across the LV and RV. Subtracting this value from the systolic blood pressure of 120 mmHg will yield a PA systolic pressure of 18 mmHg.

20. **Answer: A.**

   The image shows a still frame with continuous wave Doppler obtained from the base. The continuous wave is across the pulmonary valve. The systolic velocity is not increased, hence ruling out severe pulmonary valve stenosis. The diastolic wave above the baseline shows a rapidly decelerating waveform. This is suggestive of severe pulmonary valve regurgitation, which is a sequela of her surgery in infancy.

21. **Answer: A.**

   The LA pressure can be calculated with the following equation:

   LA pressure = (PFO velocity)^2 × 4 + right atrial pressure.

   Hence LA pressure during systole is $(2.7)^2$ × 4 + 8 = 37 mmHg. Similarly, LA pressure during diastole is $(0.9)^2$ × 4 + 8 = 11 mmHg.

22. **Answer: C.**

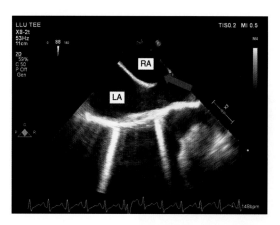

   The transesophageal echocardiography from the base shows the RA and LA with a defect in the superior portion of the atrial septum. This is suggestive of sinus venosus ASD.

23. **Answer: B.**

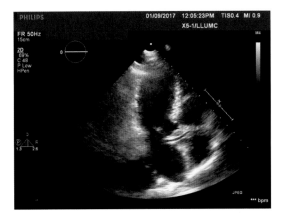

The image shows a tube-like structure that is seen to arise from the right side and is coursing toward the left side. The image is an anterior cut as the aorta is seen and hence this is an anomalous left circumflex coronary artery from the right sinus. The coronary sinus will be visible when the transducer is tilted posteriorly.

24. **Answer: C.**

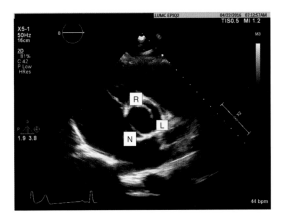

The image is a short axis view of the aortic valve from a TTE. It shows a bicuspid aortic valve with fused right and left coronary cusps. R = right coronary cusp, L = left coronary cusp, N = non coronary cusp.

25. **Answer: D.**

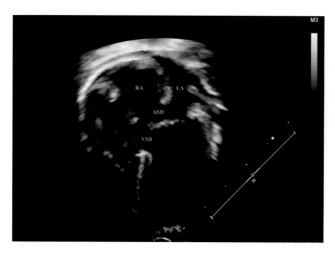

The image is a four-chamber apical view with apex down. As the labels show the patient has an ostium primum ASD and a perimembranous VSD, which constitute a complete trioventricular septal defect.

26. **Answer: B.**

The peak systolic velocity of the flow is 4.7 m/sec. The systolic gradient between aorta and PA is $4V^2$, which is $4.7 \times 4.7 \times 4 = 88$ mmHg. Subtracting 88 from the systemic systolic blood pressure of 118 mmHg yields 30 mmHg, which is the systolic PA pressure.

27. **Answer: A.**

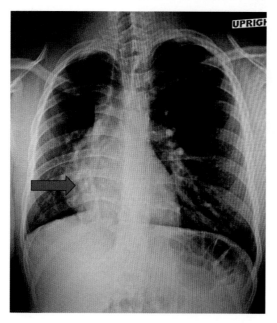

The blue arrow points to a sickle-shaped tube-like structure that is seen entering the liver. This is called scimitar (sickle) syndrome.

28. **Answer: C.**

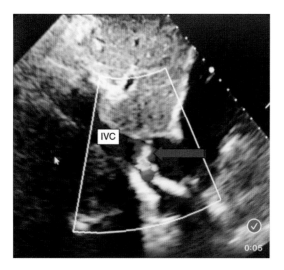

The subcostal view shows a long axis of the IVC with abnormal flow. This flow is due to the anomalous connection of the pulmonary vein into the IVC.

The blue arrow points to flow from the abnormal pulmonary vein connection into the IVC. This anomalous connection gives rise to the scimitar syndrome.

29. **Answer: D.**

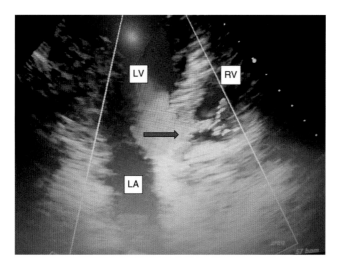

The image is an apical view with anterior tilt. It shows the perimembranous area with flow from LV into RV in systole. This is indicative of perimembranous VSD. A posterior VSD is seen when the transducer is tilted posteriorly. A supracristal VSD sits below the pulmonary valve and a muscular VSD is seen in the muscular septum. The distinction between a perimembranous VSD and a supracristal VSD can be made easily with a short axis image of the ventricles. A perimembranous VSD will be seen around the 10 o'clock position while a supracristal VSD is seen at the 1 o'clock position.

30. **Answer: B.**
    The peak systolic velocity of the continuous wave Doppler is about 6 m/sec. This translates to a LV–RV pressure gradient of 144 mmHg. Systolic blood pressure is 121 mmHg. Subtracting 121 from 144 (144 – 121 = 23) will yield systolic PA pressure, which is 23 mmHg. This is in the normal range for this patient.

27

Questions

1. The diagram shows the length of a sarcomere at rest, after contraction, and after forced increase in filling pressure or preload. The systolic strain is:

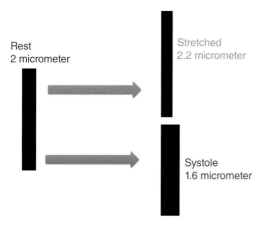

Rest
2 micrometer

Stretched
2.2 micrometer

Systole
1.6 micrometer

    A. −20% or −0.2
    B. +20% or +0.2
    C. ±27%
    D. −27%

2. In the example from Question 2, if the duration of systole was 0.25 s, the average systolic strain rate is:
    A. −0.8/s
    B. +0.8/s
    C. 0.5/s
    D. 1.25/s

Echocardiography Board Review: 600 Multiple Choice Questions with Discussion, Third Edition.
Ramdas G. Pai and Padmini Varadarajan.
© 2025 John Wiley & Sons Ltd. Published 2025 by John Wiley & Sons Ltd.

3. The diastolic strain in the example in Question 1 is:
   A. +0.25
   B. −0.25
   C. +0.1
   D. −0.1

4. During diastole, the left ventricle (LV) was overfilled increasing its volume, and sarcomeric length increased to 2.2 µm from 2 µm. The strain corresponds to:
   A. +10%
   B. −10%
   C. +37.5%
   D. −37.5%

5. Given that at rest diastole is twice as long as systole, in the example in Question 1, this strain rate is numerically greater:
   A. Systolic
   B. Diastolic

6. This is a patient with Class III heart failure with reduced ejection fraction (HFrEF) of nonischemic etiology on optimal medical management. This LV M mode suggests:

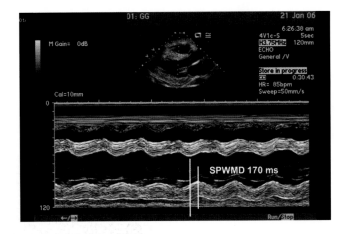

   A. Cardiac amyloid
   B. Increased LV size
   C. LV mechanical dyssynchrony
   D. LV scar

7. This is a tissue Doppler-derived mitral annular displacement against time curve – medial annulus in red and lateral annulus in yellow. The onsets, peak apical directed displacement, and annular ascent are shown. The pattern shown:

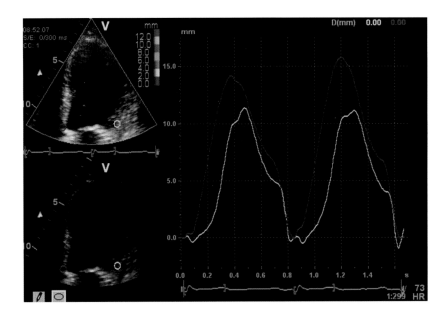

   A. Is normal

   B. Shows delayed LV lateral wall contraction

   C. Shows delayed septal wall contraction

   D. None of the above

8. In the example in Question 7, the long axis length of the LV is 90 mm in end diastole and the LV apex did not move up in relation to the transducer, so annular decent amounts to long axis shortening of the corresponding wall. LV septal (S) and lateral (L) wall strains are:

   A. $S = -17\%$, $L = -13\%$

   B. $S = 17\%$, $L = 13\%$

   C. Both $= 15\%$

9. In the example in Question 7:

   A. Septal and lateral wall strains are normal

   B. Lateral wall is abnormal

   C. Septum is abnormal

10. Tissue Doppler velocity profiles of medial (yellow) and lateral (green) mitral annuli are shown here. This is suggestive of:

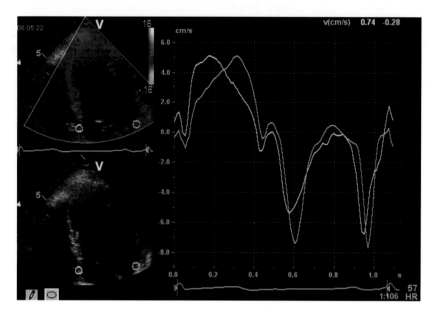

A. Good systolic and diastolic synchrony of LV
B. Delayed LV lateral wall contraction
C. Delayed septal wall contraction
D. Diastolic asynchrony only

11. This tracing represents the strain curves of LV septal (yellow) and lateral (green) wall bases. You can draw this conclusion:

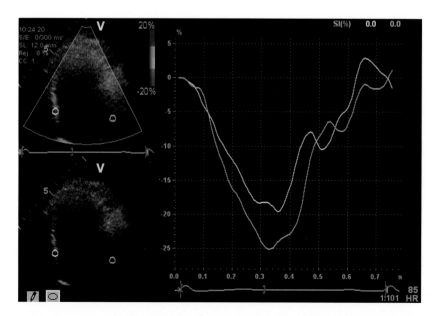

A. Normal septal but impaired LV lateral wall systolic strain
B. Normal systolic strains but septal wall asynchrony
C. Abnormal strains and abnormal wall synchrony

12. Flows in left ventricular outflow tract (LVOT) and right ventricular outflow tract (RVOT) with the timings of their onset in relation to the onset of QRS complex (137 and 81 ms respectively) are shown in this patient with nonischemic dilated cardiomyopathy. You can draw this conclusion:

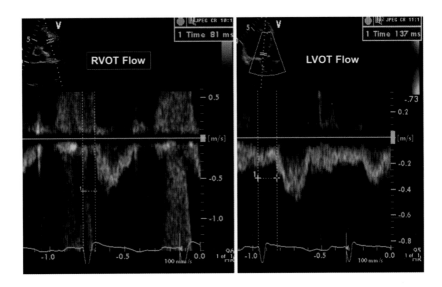

A. There is a lengthening of both LV and right ventricular (RV) preejection periods
B. There is an increase in interventricular delay
C. Both of the above

13. In the example in Question 12, you can draw this additional hemodynamic observation:
A. Reduced LV stroke volume
B. Reduced RV stroke volume
C. Both of the above
D. Neither of the above

14. In this image the arrows indicate:

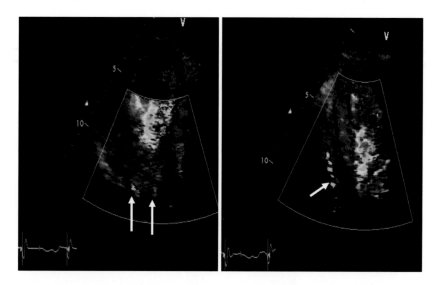

   A. Tissue Doppler velocities
   B. Coronary arteries
   C. Coronary sinus branches
   D. Artifact

15. The mitral flow by continuous wave is shown in a patient with biventricular pacemaker. The programmed atrioventricular (AV) delay is 200 ms. You can take this action to optimize LV filling:

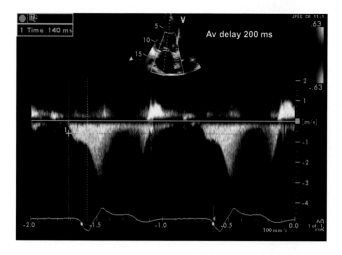

   A. Lengthen AV delay
   B. Shorten AV delay
   C. Change to VVI pacing
   D. None of the above

16–20. Match the schematics of these strain patterns with these possible diagnoses:
- A. Normal
- B. LV apical aneurysm
- C. Apical infarct
- D. Hypertrophic cardiomyopathy with asymmetric upper septal and anterior basal hypertrophy
- E. Cardiac amyloid
- F. Cardiac sarcoid
- G. Nonischemic cardiomyopathy with an ejection fraction (EF) of 20%

16.

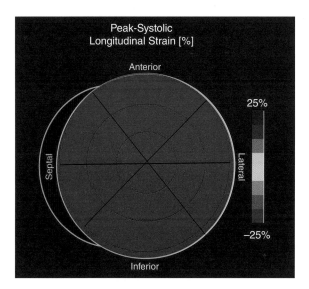

17.

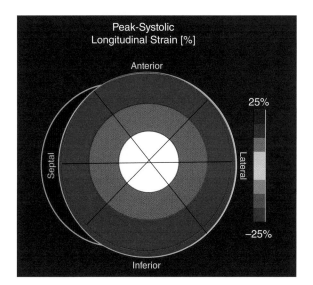

18.

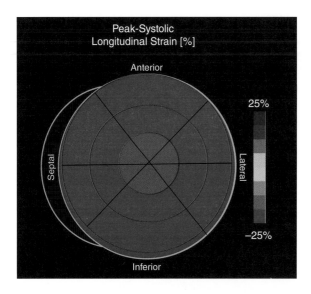

19.

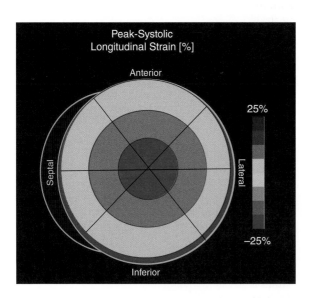

20.

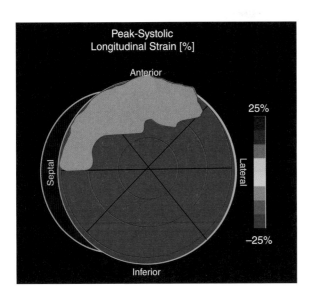

21–30. Match these properties of strain imaging techniques with the technique:
   A. Tissue Doppler strain imaging
   B. Speckle tracking strain imaging
   C. Both of the above

21. Need for high-quality imaging

22. Angle dependent

23. High frame rate requirement

24. Higher temporal resolution

25. Good for LV longitudinal strain

26. Good for LV circumferential and radial strain

27. More reproducible

28. Enables analysis of LV rotational mechanism

29. Higher vendor variability

30. 3D strain acquisition possible

31. Systolic longitudinal strain is a negative value and is around −20%. The circumferential strain of the LV in systole is:
   A. Positive
   B. Negative
   C. Does not exist

32. The systolic radial strain of the LV is:
    A. Positive
    B. Negative
    C. Neither of the above

33. The LV rotational strain is normally in the range of:
    A. 0 degree
    B. 5 degrees
    C. 15 degrees
    D. 30 degrees

34. The normal RV free wall strain obtained from an oblique apical view is:
    A. 18–23%
    B. 24–35%
    C. 36–50%

Answers for Chapter 27

1. **Answer: A.**
   −20% or −0.2. The absolute shortening of the sarcomere was 0.4 μm, that is, 20% shortening from baseline. As it is shorter in systole, strain is negative.

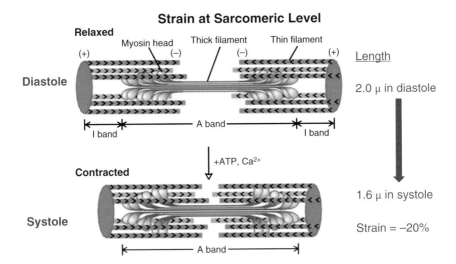

2. **Answer: A.**
   −0.8/s. Strain rate = strain/time; i.e., 0.2/0.25 s = 0.8/s.

3. **Answer: A.**
   +0.25 or +25%. Increase in length from systole/systolic length = 0.4 μm/1.6 μm = 0.25 or 25% and positive as the sarcomere lengthened.

4. **Answer: A.**
   +10%. As the length increased, strain is positive; the lengthening was 10% from baseline diastolic length.

5. **Answer: A.**
   Systolic, because of the longer duration of diastole. In this example diastolic strain rate is 0.25/0.5 s = 0.5/s and systolic strain rate is 0.2/0.25 s = 0.8/s. But at faster heart rates this reverses and diastolic strain rate becomes considerably higher (because diastole becomes disproportionately shorter compared to systole), thus exposing early myocardial dysfunction earlier through diastolic dysfunction.

6. **Answer: C.**
   LV mechanical dyssynchrony. Note that the septum thickens first followed by the LV posterior wall after a delay of 170 ms. In this LV septal–posterior wall mechanical delay, anything > 130 ms is abnormal. Left ventricular end diastolic diameter (LVEDD) is 45 mm (not dilated) and there is no thinning, suggesting a scar. The patient has LV hypertrophy and cardiac amyloid is a possibility if there are other signs such as low QRS voltage or Q waves.

7. **Answer: B.**

   Delayed LV lateral wall contraction. Note that the onset of LV lateral wall contraction is delayed compared to the septum by about 130 ms. As a matter of fact, the LV lateral wall paradoxically lengthens when the septum starts to contract. Also, the peak descent of the lateral wall is late by about 120 ms as well compared to the septum. This is an example of extreme LV septolateral dyssynchrony – any value > 40 ms is abnormal. Normally all walls contract and relax synchronously, thus optimizing mechanical efficiency.

8. **Answer: A.**

   S = −17%, L = −13%. The length of each wall is 90 mm. S descended or shortened by 15 mm (from the tracing), giving a S strain of −15/90 = −17%. Similarly, L strain is −12/90 = −13%. This is not segmental but is for the entire wall – all three segments together.

9. **Answer: B.**

   The lateral wall is abnormal. Normal mitral annular plane systolic excursion (MAPSE) is between 15 and 20 mm – generally the least in the septum and the highest in the lateral wall. Note that the lengths of these walls being 90–100 mm, this translates to a longitudinal LV shortening of 17–20% in normal individuals – normal values for longitudinal LV strain!

10. **Answer: B.**

    Delayed LV lateral wall contraction. Note that the peak velocity in the lateral annulus is delayed compared to the medial annulus. This is an LV septolateral delay of 150 ms, a marker of severe LV mechanical dyssynchrony. There is a fairly good diastolic synchrony in this patient.

11. **Answer: B.**

    Normal systolic strains, but there is septal wall asynchrony. Note that the septal and lateral wall strains are −20 and 25%, respectively, which are normal. But the timing of the peak negative strain of the septal base is delayed compared to that of the lateral wall.

12. **Answer: C.**

    Both A and B. The preejection period (PEP) is measured from the onset of QRS to onset of ejection. This is normally < 100 ms for the LV and < 70 ms for the RV. In this patient both are prolonged, indicating both LV and RV systolic dysfunction. PEP is composed of electromechanical delay and isovolumic contraction time. In addition, the onset of LV ejection is markedly delayed compared to that of the RV (137 − 81 = 56 ms), a measure of interventricular dyssynchrony.

13. **Answer: C.**

    Both. Note the LVOT peak velocity is 40 cm/s and its duration is 0.2 s; assuming the signal is triangular (triangular approximation), the area under the curve (base multiplied by height, divided by 2) or its time velocity integral is (40 cm/s × 0.2 s)/2 = 4 cm. In normal individuals it is around 20 cm, which corresponds to a stroke volume of about 70 cc assuming an average LVOT area of 3.5 cm². In the absence of aortic or mitral regurgitation, the LV and RV stroke volume have to be equal. Also note that the second ejection signal in the LVOT has a lower velocity and duration compared to the first, despite being in sinus rhythm – in other words, this patient has Doppler equivalent of pulsus alternans as well.

14. **Answer: C.**
    Coronary sinus branches. Note that the flow is blue (away from the transducer and the apex or toward the LV base and it is in systole). This is the direction of flow in the branches of the coronary sinus. This best shown by color flow power mode (not variance mode). Flow in the coronary arteries is toward the apex and will be red, and will also be mostly in diastole.

15. **Answer: B.**
    Shorten AV delay. Note that this patient has marked presystolic diastolic mitral regurgitation (MR) and the duration of this diastolic MR is 140 ms. Shortening the programmed AV delay by this amount to 60 ms would eliminate diastolic MR. This diastolic MR is occurring because of atrial relaxation, which produces a suction effect by the left atrium. The goal is to time the atrial systole just before ventricular systole.

16. **Answer**
    Normal. All 16 segments have a strain between −18% and −25% uniformly.

17. **Answer**
    LV apical infarct. Markedly reduced strain in apex extending to the mid segments consistent with a large wraparound left anterior descending artery.

18. **Answer**
    LV apical aneurysm. Paradoxic lengthening of apical segments with LV systole.

19. **Answer**
    Cardiac amyloid. Cherry on top appearance due to diminished function in the bases and preserved function at the apex.

20. **Answer**
    Hypertrophic cardiomyopathy with asymmetric upper septal and anterior basal hypertrophy. Reduced strain in hypertrophied segments due to a combination of myocardial disarray, fibrosis and ischemia.
    In nonischemic cardiomyopathy, the longitudinal strain would be reduced fairly uniformly. In cardiac sarcoid, strain reductions and aneurysms tend to be in noncoronary distributions – typically basal septum, mid-septal aneurysms, etc.

21. **Answer**
    Need for high-quality imaging: Speckle tracking as you need good 2D images with visible speckles throughout systole and have to make sure that tissue tracking is reliable.

22. **Answer**
    Angle dependent: Tissue Doppler. This is the property of Doppler.

23. **Answer**
    High frame rate requirement: Both for adequate temporal resolution.

24. **Answer**
    Higher temporal resolution: Tissue Doppler has a higher temporal resolution up to 160 Hz and is better for timing purposes.

25. **Answer**
    Good for LV longitudinal strain: Both.

26. **Answer**
    Good for LV circumferential and radial strain: Only speckle tracking as it is not angle dependent.

27. **Answer**
    More reproducible: Tissue Doppler.

28. **Answer**
    Enables analysis of LV rotational mechanism: Speckle tracking because of nonangle dependency and oblique planes needed.

29. **Answer**
    Higher vendor variability: Speckle tracking because of varying proprietary analysis algorithms and speckle definitions and its reliability.

30. **Answer**
    3D strain acquisition possible: Speckle tracking only, not Tissue Doppler.

31. **Answer: B.**
    Negative. As the circumference of the LV gets less during systole, it is negative. The numerical values (without a sign) are larger for the endocardium compared to mid-wall and epicardium. Numerical value of endocardial circumferential strain would be the same as LV fractional shortening (FS) which is (LVEDD – LVESD)/LVEDD, as Pi in both numerator and denominator cancel out and the ratio of change in circumference over initial circumference would be the same as the ratio of change in LV diameter over initial diameter.

32. **Answer: A.**
    Positive. It is nothing but fractional thickening of the LV wall during systole; normally it thickens by 30–50% compared to diastolic thickness.
    This figure simplifies the concepts of different types of LV strain.

Types of LV Strain

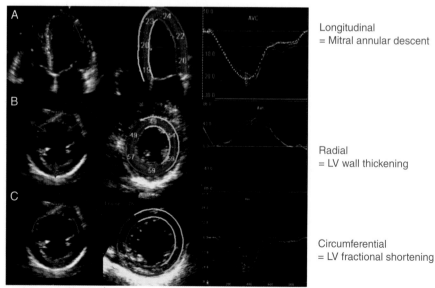

Longitudinal
= Mitral annular descent

Radial
= LV wall thickening

Circumferential
= LV fractional shortening

33. **Answer: C.**

15 degrees. Normally, viewed from the apex, the LV base rotates about 5 degrees clockwise (red) and apex rotates about 10 degrees counterclockwise (blue) – net rotation is 15 degrees and it is a wringing motion.

Rotational Strain Imaging from a Normal Subject

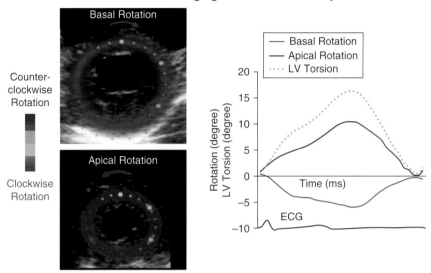

34. **Answer: B.**

24–35%. The RV free wall strain is greater than that of the LV. Easy way to remember is: Tricuspid annular plane systolic excursion (TAPSE) is 18–25 mm (more than MAPSE) and the RV free wall length is 6–7 cm (less than LV free wall length).

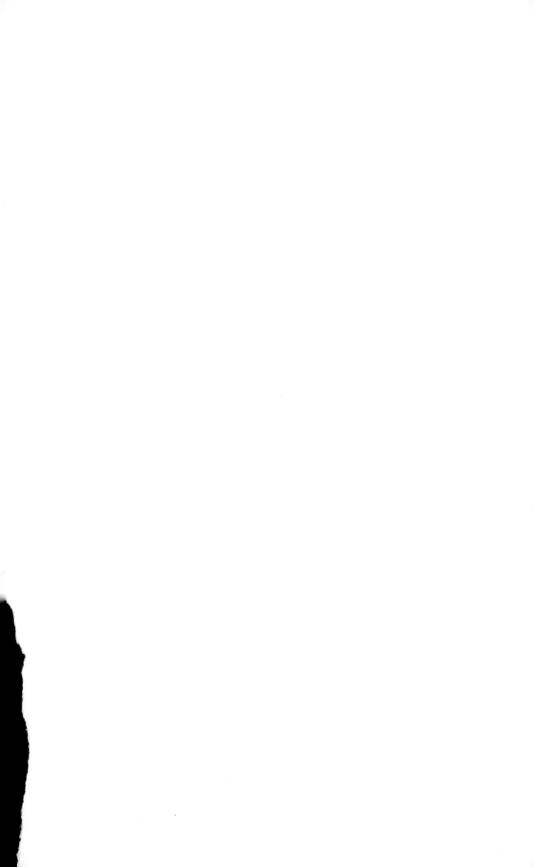